Study Guide
for

Human Communication Disorders

Study Guide
for

Shames · Wiig · Secord
Human Communication Disorders
An Introduction
Fifth Edition

Prepared by
William Culbertson
Northern Arizona University

Allyn and Bacon
Boston · London · Toronto · Sydney · Tokyo · Singapore

Table of Contents

INTRODUCTION to the STUDENTS' GUIDE

This students' guide accompanies the text, *Human Communication Disorders: an Introduction* (5th Edition), by George Shames, Wayne Secord and Elisabeth Wiig. You may use it as a "study map" to help you, the undergraduate student, organize your intellectual course through an introduction to communication disorders. The field of communication and its disorders is vast and any text must cover a large territory. The undergraduate student who is contemplating a career in this rewarding field needs a comprehensive overview of its many aspects. Careful study in your survey class will enable you not only to decide if a career in speech-language pathology, audiology or speech and hearing science is for you, but it may also pique a little interest in a focus area for future study.

This students' guide is arranged in successive steps to encourage students' assimilation of the material. The steps guide students from general to particular in their study, and end with a self test to facilitate review.

A **Chapter Summary**, in narrative form, begins each section of the guide. Chapter summaries allow students to get a general idea of the material contained in text chapters. Summaries might also be a good way to review or "warm up" just before a test. Read the paragraph summary and the learner outcomes listed at the beginning of each chapter. They will give you the idea of what material is contained in the text and of what the expectations of the student may be.

Critical Concepts form the next section of the guide chapters. Before you begin a text section, look over the *italicized* "Critical Concepts." You will notice that these concepts are organized according to the major text chapter headings. The Critical Concept items are selected to alert and orient students to the major issues developed by text authors. To respond to the Critical Concept items, you have to read the text material for each heading. Read the text carefully, and ask yourself questions about certain concepts presented therein. There are spaces in this guide for you to write your answers for future reference. For many students, the act of writing down concepts in an organized form is a great help in analyzing and synthesizing information. You may need extra paper to rewrite or consolidate your responses to the critical concept items. Your goal should be to answer those items without returning to the text for reference.

The **Self Test** section at the end of each chapter allows you to see if you really have the ideas for each text chapter "down" before you go into the "real test." Each self test section contains True/False and Multiple Choice questions to round out the experience of chapter study. Those who are interested in essay questions may infer them from the critical concept sections. You may take these self tests alone or team up with a study group. If you discover you have missed any material, your next step is to review those areas. The answers are in the back of the book.

Good luck and good studying!

Study Guide
for

Human Communication Disorders

CHAPTER GUIDES

Chapter One Students' Guide

The Professions of Speech-Language Pathology and Audiology

Fred Spahr and Russ Malone

Chapter Summary

The purpose of this chapter is to introduce students to the fields of Audiology and Speech-Language Pathology. These fields deal with one of the most basic human functions: communication. Like the other chapters in the text, the first chapter begins with the personal views of the chapter's authors, both past presidents of the American Speech-Language and Hearing Association. There follows a discussion of the characteristics of a profession, any profession, relating nine attributes that qualify speech-language pathology and audiology as professions in the truest sense. The incidence of communicative disorders in the United States establishes the relevance and need for professionals who specialize in the study and treatment of communication disorders. The next three sections present "What Do They Do?" descriptions of audiology, speech-language pathology and speech, language and hearing science. Authors discuss branches of the profession and relate them to everyday life. This is followed by discussions of employment opportunities, personal attributes and professional preparation requirements. The last section of the chapter describes professional organizations related to speech-language pathology and audiology in general with the focus on the American Speech-Language and Hearing Association in particular.

Student Outcomes

After reading this chapter, the students should be able to do the following:

☞ Apply nine characteristics of a profession to the fields of speech-language pathology and audiology.

☞ Relate the prevalence of communication disorders to the need for trained professionals in the fields of speech-language pathology and audiology.

☞ Briefly describe the professional activities of the speech-language pathologist.

☞ Briefly describe the professional activities of the audiologist.

☞ List three personal attributes required for a professional in communication disorders.

☞   List the educational and practicum requirements for certification by the American Speech-Language and Hearing Association.

☞   Identify two professional organizations serving the interests of speech-language pathologists and audiologists.

☞   List three professional activities of the speech, language and hearing scientist.

☞   Apply three types of credentialing to the professions of speech-language pathology and audiology.

Critical Concepts

Section:

Are audiology and Speech-language pathology professions?

Concept:

There is a tacit acknowledgment among professional and legal entities that speech-language pathology and audiology are independent professions.

Show how speech-language pathology or audiology demonstrates the following characteristics:

1.   Cuts across a comprehensive complex aspect of living but has a basic centralizing unit:

2.   Has several aspects which can be ordered or organized:

3.   Draws from other fields, but has its own distinct body of research theory and experience:

4.   Specifies its own areas of concentration and function:

5.   Determines its standards and is continues to raise the standards of its members:

6.   Describes and enforces a code of ethics:

7.   Systematically informs the public:

8.   Provides for a medium of exchange among its members:

9.   Relates to other professions on an organizational level:

Section:

Do communication problems constitute a major problem?

Concept:

Communicative disorders impact a large number of Americans. See also: introduction to section V.

1.   According to Bello (1995) what proportion of Americans have communicative disorders?

2.   What is the economic impact of communicative disorders in the United States?

Section:

What do Audiologists do?

Concept: *Audiologists are hearing health care professionals.*

1.   Briefly describe the professional activities of the audiologist:

2.   What role does the audiologist play in prevention of hearing disorders?

3.   What aspects of hearing loss does the audiologist assess?

4.   What tools does the audiologist use in rehabilitation?

5.   Why is counseling an important part of the audiologist's role?

6.   Name some important rehabilitation team members for people with hearing disorders.

Section:

What do speech-language pathologists do?

Concept:

Speech-language pathologists have a wide scope of practice for individuals who have receptive or expressive communicative disorders.

1.   Describe five types of speech or language disorders that may be ameliorated through the services of a speech-language pathologist.

2.   How do speech-language pathologists *prevent* speech-language problems?

3.   Name seven members of an *ideal* treatment team on which might also serve an audiologist and a speech-language pathologist.

    A.

    B.

    C.

    D.

    E.

    F.

    G..

Section:

The speech, language and hearing scientists.

Concept:

Speech, language and hearing scientists continue development of the body of knowledge about human communication and its disorders.

1.   List five activities of speech, language and hearing scientists:

2.   Where are speech, language and hearing scientists employed?

Section:

Career and Job Opportunities

Concept:

Employment of speech-language pathologists and audiologists should increase at a higher rate than that for all occupations through the year 2005.

1.   Give five reasons for an optimistic outlook for employment of professionals in the speech-language pathology and audiology.

A.

B.

C.

D.

E.

2. Name five types of professional activities in which speech-language pathologists and audiologists may engage.

    A.

    B.

    C.

    D.

    E.

Section:

Attributes and Requirements

Concept:

Those who choose caring professions should possess certain personal attributes. The educational and practical preparation may begin in high school but must continue through graduate school.

1. List four personal skills that may be required of a professional in speech-language pathology or audiology.

    A.

    B.

    C.

    D.

2.   Describe the educational requirements for the independent practitioner in speech-language pathology or audiology.

Section:

Credentialing

Concept:

Individuals may be certified and licensed by professional and governmental boards. Institutions may be accredited by professional organizations.

1.   Describe the difference between certification and licensure.

Section:

Associations

Concept:

Audiologists and speech-language pathologists may belong to several regional, state national and international associations.

1. What is the foremost association for speech-language pathologists and audiologists in the United States?

2. Name one (each) other United States professional association to which speech-language pathologists or audiologists may belong.

3. List nine activities of professional associations that may benefit their members.

    A.

    B.

    C.

    D.

    E.

    F.

    G.

    H.

    I.

Section:

Rewards

Concept:

The rewards of practice in speech-language pathology or audiology are personal as well as monetary.

1. What rewards might you personally derive from a career in speech-language pathology or audiology? (You may write your answer on a separate sheet or simply discuss this concept with your classmates.)

Critical Terms

Define the following terms, using your text as a reference:

o   Profession

o   Identification

o   Articulation

o   Credentialing

o   Licensure

o   Prevention

o   Aural Rehabilitation

o   Speech-Language Pathology

o   Assessment

o   Certification

o   Ethics

o   Team

o   Aphasia

o   Prevalence

Chapter One Self Test

True/False

1. The titles, "Speech-Language Pathologist" and "Audiologist " describe the same professionals.
    True
    False
2. Most professions describe and enforce their own ethical codes.
    True
    False
3. Once professional standards are established, they remain never change.
    True
    False
4. Communication disorders have no economic impact in the United States..
    True
    False
5. Audiologists are health care professionals who specialize in swallowing disorders.
    True
    False
6. Hearing loss can be prevented.
    True
    False
7. Audiological assessment can only be performed with adult patients
    True
    False
8. A hearing aid can cure a hearing loss.
    True
    False
9. A rehabilitation team directs the person with the hearing loss.
    True
    False
10. Speech-Language Pathologists provide remedial services to people with voice disorders..
    True
    False
11. Dysphagia is a loss or impairment of language following brain damage.
    True
    False

12. Speech-Language Pathologists help people whose voices are too hoarse.
> True
> False

13. Articulation disorders may distract the listener.
> True
> False

14. A speech or language disorder may signal the onset of a "stroke."
> True
> False

15. All speech scientists may be employed by private laboratories
> True
> False

16. Disordered articulation may be associated with a medical condition.
> True
> False

17. The prevalence of communication disorders is increasing in the United States.
> True
> False

18. In 1995, over one half of speech-language pathologists worked in schools.
> True
> False

19. The Master's degree is needed to practice Audiology or Speech-Language Pathology.
> True
> False

20. Professional Licensure in all 50 of the United States is managed by the American Speech-Language and Hearing Association..
> True
> False

Multiple Choice

1. Which of the following is *not* characteristic of a profession?
   a. A profession is a highly paid employment opportunity.
   b. A profession delineates its areas of function.
   c. A profession determines and continues to raise standards of competence of its members.
   d. A profession develops a distinct body of information.

2.   Which organization represents both speech-language pathologists and audiologists?
    a.   The American Speech-Language and Hearing Association
    b.   The Acoustic Society of America
    c.   The American Academy of Audiology
    d.   The Council of Supervisors in Speech-Language Pathology and Audiology

3.   Speech-Language and Hearing scientists may be employed at...
    a.   Universities.
    b.   Private Laboratories.
    c.   Government Agencies.
    d.   All of the above.

4.   Which of the following people are regularly exposed to potentially damaging noise?
    a.   Librarians
    b.   Swimmers
    c.   Home Owners Doing Yard Work
    d.   Ministers

5.   Which of the following is way to prevent hearing loss?
    a.   Education
    b.   Wearing Hearing Protection
    c.   Avoiding Ototoxic Drugs
    d.   All of the Above

6.   The effects of hearing loss on normal language development will be minimized if...
    a.   a child is male.
    b.   a child is from a high income family.
    c.   the hearing loss is identified early.
    d.   English is the primary language.

7.   Audiologists are employed by industry to...
    a.   ensure compliance with OSHA standards.
    b.   establishing prevention and early detection programs.
    c.   dispensing hearing aids in the workplace.
    d.   all of the Above.

8.   A conscious effort to simulate a hearing loss when one does not exist is called...
    a.   malingering.
    b.   a Conductive Hearing Loss.
    c.   sensorineural Hearing Loss.
    d.   audition.

9.   A physician who specialized in diseases of the ear is called a/an...
    a.   Gastroenterologist
    b.   Otologist.
    c.   Urologist.
    d.   Neurologist.

10. Which two speech sounds might cause confusion for speech readers?
    a. /s/ and /h/.
    b. /p/ and /b/.
    c. /l/ and /m/.
    d. /f/ and /p/.

11. Which of the following has the most important place on a rehabilitation team along with a Speech-Language Pathologist and an Audiologist?
    a. Medical Doctor
    b. The Person with the Hearing Loss and Her Family
    c. Psychologist
    d. Educational Specialist

12. Difficulty with expression and comprehension of language across all the language channels is...
    a. dysarthria.
    b. aphasia.
    c. dysphagia.
    d. dysgraphia.

13. Voice disorders may include...
    a. breathiness.
    b. hoarseness.
    c. low Pitch.
    d. all of the above.

14. The most effective means of preventing Speech and language problems in children is...
    a. information and Counseling.
    b. therapy.
    c. diet.
    d. surgery.

15. Which of the following might need the services of an Audiologist?
    a. crack babies
    b. yard workers
    c. rock musicians
    d. all of the above

Chapter Two Students' Guide

Development of Communication, Language and Speech

Robert E. Owens, Jr.

Chapter Summary

Chapter Two examines the growth of communication in children, from birth through the school age years. Underlying the material is the basic assumption that there is a difference between *Language* and *Communication*. While language is one way in which we communicate, it is not the only way. The author describes the difference. Theories relating to the normal development of speech, language, and communication as interrelated, yet speak in terms of separate processes. The dimensions of speech, language, and communication are examined, and normal developmental sequences are discussed.

Student Outcomes

After reading this chapter, students should be able to do the following:

☞ Define and differentiate between the terms SPEECH, LANGUAGE, and COMMUNICATION.

☞ Discus the normal developmental sequences of speech, language, and communication skills.

☞ Identify the five distinct, but interrelated components of language including: SYNTAX, MORPHOLOGY, PHONOLOGY, SEMANTICS, and, PRAGMATICS.

☞ Detail the various components of speech, language, and communication.

☞ Describe the major differences in the language, speech, and communication abilities of infants and toddlers, preschoolers, and school-aged children/adults.

☞ Outline the early development of the speech mechanism and speech production.

Critical Concepts

Section

Communication

Critical Concept

Communication is a process of exchange, uniquely developed in human beings. It includes, but is not limited to, the use of language.

1.   Write the Owens' (text author) definition of *Communication* in the space below.

2.   The text presents examples of *paralinguistic, nonlinguistic* and *metalinguistic* communication. Write two other examples of each in the space below.

   a. *Paralinguistic Communication:*

   b. *Nonlinguistic Communication:*

   c. *Metalinguistic Communication:*

Section:

Development of Communication

Critical Concept:

A predictable sequence of communicative development begins at birth.

1. Describe how an infant's mother (or care giver) enhances communicative development.

2. What is the earliest form of communication normally seen in an infant? Is this a nonlinguistic, linguistic, paralinguistic or metalinguistic form?

3. Using the text as a guide, trace the development of different communication components from birth to age eight.

    a. Nonlinguistic Communication:

    b. Linguistic Communication:

    c. Paralinguistic Communication:

    d. Metalinguistic Communication:

Section:

Language:

Critical Concept:

Language is defined as a..."Socially shared code or conventional system for representing concepts through the use of arbitrary symbols and rule governed combinations of those symbols." *(Bloom, L., and Lahey, M.. (1978).* Language Disorders and Language Development. *New York: Wiley).*

1. Look the word *Language* up in three dictionaries and write the principal definitions below. How do those definitions compare with the one presented in the text?

    a.

    b.

    c.

2. In your own words, apply the five components of Bloom's and Lahey's language definition to spoken communication.

     a. Socially-Shared

     b. Code or Conventional System

     c. Representation of Concepts

     d. Symbols

     e. Rule-Governed Combinations

3. What is the difference between *linguistic competence* and *linguistic performance*?

Section:

Components of Language

Critical concept:

There are five major components of language. Researchers have identified predictable milestones for their development in "Toddler," Preschool, School-Age and Adult years.

1. In the space below, define each of the five components of language. Tell how each is distinct from the others. Then tell how each is similar to the others.

Syntax

Morphology

Phonology

Semantics

Pragmatics

Section:

Language Development

Critical Concept:

Different children will develop different skills at different times and rates, but the general sequence is predictable. This holds true for the five components of language.

1. For each age categories below, describe the general sequence of development for each of the five language components.

    a. Toddler:

        I. Syntax

        ii. Morphology

        iii. Phonology

        iv. Semantics

        v. Pragmatics

    b. Preschooler:

        I. Syntax

ii. Morphology

iii. Phonology

iv. Semantics

v. Pragmatics

vi.   Preschool Language Learning Strategies: *Briefly describe what the author means by the following language learning strategies:*

   (1) Language Learned Through Conversation:

   (2) Form Follows Function:

   (3) Bootstrapping:

   (4) Active Involvement:

24

(5) Complexity And Utterance Length Related:

(6) Avoid Exceptions:

(7) Word Order is a Guide:

(8) Avoid Deviation from or Interruption of Standard Word Order:

(9) Care givers Modify Conversation to maximize Child Participation:

(10) All Aspects of Language Are Intertwined in Development:

c. School Aged and Adult:

    I. Syntax

    ii. Morphology

    iii. Phonology

    iv. Semantics

    v. Pragmatics

Section:

Speech

Critical Concept:

Speech is a modality of communication in which the symbols are sequences of sounds made by modifying the flow of air from the lungs through the mouth and nose. Speech sounds may be organized in phoneme groups by using a "traditional approach" or one of several distinctive feature systems.

1. How many modalities of communication can you think of besides speech? Do any of them use sound?

2. What is a phoneme? Why is a phoneme called a *group* of sounds?

3. What is an allophone? How many allophones of a voiceless bilabial plosive (/ π /) can you make?

4. What is the *International Phonetic Alphabet* and why do we use it?

5. If you have access to an internet browser, download:

   http://www.arts.gla.ac.uk/IPA

6. Describe the characteristics of speech in the following developmental stages:

   a. Newborn:

   b. 2-3 months:

   c. 4-6 months:

   d. 6-10 months:

   e. 11-14 months:

7. Write in the probable phonological process involved when a child says...

   a. "Bacuum" for "Vacuum"

   b. "Sue" for "Shoe"

   c. "Tuttie" for "Cookie"

Critical Terms

Define the following terms, using your text as a reference:

o　　　Language

o　　　Nonlinguistic

o　　　Joint Action

o　　　Phonology

o　　　Morpheme

o　　　Underextension

o　　　Conjoining

o　　　Morphophonemic Changes

o　　　Speech

o　　　Metalinguistic

o　　　Joint Reference

o　　　Syntax

o　　　Semantics

o　　　Phoneme

o　　　Similes

o　　　Turnabout

o　　　Bootstrapping

o　　　Communication

o　　　Idioms

o   Morphology

o   Metaphors

o   Speech Act

o   Embedding

o   Proverbs

o   Paralinguistic

o   Babbling

o   Pragmatics

o   Overextension

o   Phonetically Consistent Forms

Chapter Two Self Test

True/False

1.   Language is a conventional system of symbols.
           True
           False

2.   In most children, communicative development is a phenomenon related to, but separate from speech development.
           True
           False

3.   *This Little Piggy* is an example of a joint action routine.
           True
           False

4.   Development of the intonation patterns in speech reflect maturation of the paralinguistic aspect of communication.
           True
           False

5.   The form or structure of a sentence is governed by syntactic rules.
           True
           False

6.   Phonological rules govern the meaning and relationships between meaning units.
           True
           False

7.   The smallest unit of grammar is an morpheme.
           True
           False

8.   Word knowledge precedes language.
           True
           False

9.   Repetition strings of the same consonant-vowel combinations, such as *bababa*, are called reduplications.
           True
           False

10.   Early words are learned receptively and then produced expressively.
           True
           False

11.   A *bound* morpheme can function independently in a sentence.
           True
           False

12. Pragmatic rules govern speech acts.
    True
    False
13. Most children have learned 90% of adult syntax by the time they have entered kindergarten.
    True
    False
14. A child's lexicon is a personal dictionary.
    True
    False
15. Native speakers of a language learn permissible rule combinations of that language.
    True
    False
16. Free morphemes are independent and can be used independently.
    True
    False
17. Most toddlers learn verbs before they learn nouns.
    True
    False
18. Many experts believe that imitation forms the roots of symbolic function.
    True
    False
19. The order of consonant acquisition can be predicted by the frequency of their usage or appearance in a child's native language.
    True
    False
20. Traditional classification of vowels is by place and manner of articulation.
    True
    False
21. Bilabial consonants are the easiest for a child to articulate.
    True
    False
22. Phonological rules govern sound distribution and sequencing.
    True
    False
23. Speech development appears related to increased control over oral muscles.
    True
    False
24. English consonants which differ only in terms of voicing are called cognates.
    True
    False

Multiple Choice

1. Communication involves the active processes of :
   a. Syntax, semantics, phonology.
   b. Place, manner, voicing.
   c. Encoding, transmitting, decoding.
   d. Intonation, stress, rate.

2. Bloom and Lahey (1978) described language as:
   a. A socially shared code.
   b. Words, sentences, and paragraphs.
   c. The native tongue of an entire country.
   d. A messaging system.

3. Which aspect of language is concerned with permissible sound combinations?
   a. Pragmatics
   b. Morphology
   d. Phonology
   e. Semantics

4. The science of word meaning is called:
   a. Syntax
   b. Semantics
   c. Pragmatics
   d. Metalinguistics

5. Linguistic meaning units are called:
   a. Morphemes
   b. Phonemes
   c. Acts
   d. Allophones

6. Small changes in speech sounds that are not sufficient to change word meaning are called:
   a. Phonemic
   b. Sound families
   c. Metalinguistic
   d. Allophonic

7. The earliest communication between care-giver and child probably involves:
   a. Guttural oral sounds
   b. Head movements and gaze patterns
   c. A shared system of symbols, signs, or actions
   d. Turn taking

8. The earliest use of verbal intentions normally appears by the:
   - a. First month of life.
   - b. Sixth month of life.
   - c. First year of life.
   - d. Second year of life.

9. Paralinguistic, nonlinguistic and metalinguistic communication makes its greatest developmental strides during which stage of life?
   - a. The sixth month.
   - b. The preschool period.
   - c. The metaphonemic stage.
   - d. The school-age.

10. A language user's underlying knowledge about a linguistic rule system may be called:
    - a. Linguistic competence.
    - b. Morphophonemic transference
    - c. Allophonic variation.
    - d. Metalinguistic relativism

11. Language use may described as :
    - a. Content
    - b. Function
    - c. Pragmatics
    - d. Form

12. Syntactic rules govern:
    - a. The order of sequential linguistic units.
    - b. The meaning of linguistic units
    - c. The list of permissible speech sounds.
    - d. Long-distance telephone rates for a region.

13. Body posture, facial expression and physical proximity are clues in which aspects of communication?
    - a. Nonlinguistic
    - b. Paralinguistic
    - c. Metalinguistic
    - d. Phonological

14. What process enables a speaker to use language knowledge to produce more language?:
    - a. Joint attention
    - b. Turn taking
    - c. Joint reference
    - d. Bootstrapping

15. What do linguists call the phonological changes that occur when speakers join certain morphemes?
    a. Semantic
    b. Bootstrapping
    c. Morphophonemic
    d. Metalinguistic
16. Adult-like use of stress of emphasis in speech is mastered by which age?
    a. Infant
    b. Toddler
    c. School-age
    d. Adult
17. Words that share identical semantic features are called...
    a. Homonyms
    b. Antonyms
    c. Synonyms
    d. Pseudonyms
18. Which speech sounds require a closed or constricted vocal tract passage?
    a. Vowels
    b. Diphthongs
    c. Monophthongs
    d. Consonants
19. Psycholinguists attempt to explain...
    a. Syntactic rules.
    b. The relationship between language form and cognitive processing.
    c. Speech articulation development.
    d. Morphological principles.
20. Which parts of speech predominate the vocabularies of most toddlers?
    a. Nouns
    b. Verbs
    c. Prepositions
    d. Adverbs
21. Subphoneme units of speech sound analysis are called:
    a. Distinctive features
    b. Lip rounding, place, and tenseness
    c. Manner, place, and voicing
    d. Free variation
22. Which of the following is an aspect of the traditional consonant phoneme classification system?
    a. Allophonic variation
    b. Strident deletion
    c. Manner of articulation
    d. Tense/lax

23.   When a child's word meaning features contain more examples than the adult meaning, they are called:
          a.   Underextensions
          b.   Overextensions
          c.   Metaextensions
          d.   Betaextensions

24.   A grammatic form that contains both a noun and a verb is called a...
          a.   Predicate
          b.   Subject
          c.   Modifier
          d.   Clause

25.   Saying "wawa " for "water" is an example of which phonological processes?
          a.   Reduplication
          b.   Assimilation
          c.   Deletion of unstressed syllables
          d.   Reduction of consonant clusters

26.   The developmental stage in which a child appears to experiment with sounds through long periods of vocalizing strings of meaningless sounds is called...
          a.   The experimenting stage
          b.   Phonotactics
          c.   Substitution
          d.   Babbling

Chapter Three Students' Guide

Anatomy and Physiology of Speech

Willard R. Zemlin

Chapter Summary

An overview of the various anatomical structures and systems involved in the production of speech and language is essential to the study of human communication and its disorders. The organs that enable human beings to communicate are located in the head, neck and trunk. To provide structure and organization to study, scientists group the anatomical structures of communication into several systems: the respiratory, phonatory, articulatory, and nervous systems. The hearing and visual systems are vital for normal signal recaption. This chapter examines the major structures of these systems and discusses their functions.

Student Outcomes

After reading this chapter students should be able to do the following:

☞ Differentiate the biological and the speech functions of the organs involved in speech production.

☞ Differentiate the anatomical components of the respiratory system, the phonatory system, the articulatory system and the nervous system.

☞ Describe the muscular functions involved in voice production and in changing in vocal pitch and loudness.

☞ Apply the physiology of the articulatory mechanism to the production of vowels and consonants

☞ Differentiate the communication roles of the central and the peripheral divisions of the human nervous system.

Critical Concepts

Section:

Introduction

Critical Concept:

Human beings communicate by adapting structures of their bodies to make the signals of language. These structures have other biological functions, but are pressed into service to perform their biosocial communicative duties. Speech structures are contained in the trunk. Although they must function in concert, scientists study them as component systems.

1. Describe the basic communicative functions of the following components of the human communication system.

    A. Lungs

    B. Larynx

    C. Tongue, Jaw, and Lip

    E. Hearing Mechanism

2.   What is *Resonance*?

3.   Describe how vowels and obstruent consonants are formed by alteration of the shape, length and patency of the vocal tract. How are sonorant consonants formed?

    A. Vowel formation:

    B. Obstruent Consonant formation:

    C. Sonorant Consonant Formation:

Section:

Respiration

Critical Concept:

The respiratory system provides pressurized air, the first requirement for normal speech. The muscles of respiration move air in and out of the system by acting on a framework of bone and cartilage. Structures of the upper respiratory tract conduct air to and from the lower respiratory function for both phonation and speech articulation. The lower respiratory tract contains the lungs and bronchial tree. These provide a vehicle for metabolic blood gas exchange and air pressure increase below the glottis for speech. Although the patterns of air flow for life breathing differ from those for speech, diseases of respiration are frequently associated with speech difficulties.

1.   The Bronchial Tree and Lungs

      A.   How is the trachea connected to the alveoli?

      B.   How do the lungs adhere to the inside of the chest wall?

2.   The Respiratory Muscles

      A.   During quiet breathing, which muscles contract: those of inhalation or those of exhalation?

      B.   What is the most important muscle of respiration and how does it function?

            I. Name:

            ii. Function:

3.   Basic Respiratory Physiology

      A.   Describe the differences between tidal volume, vital capacity and residual volume:

B.   What is the average adult tidal volume?

C.   What is the normal respiratory rate for adults?

4.   Speech Breathing:

      A.   List three differences between speech breathing and quiet respiration
            I.

            ii.

            iii.

      B.   Describe the roles of the muscles of exhalation in speech:

      C.   What is the ratio of the normal relaxation pressure for speech to that of 100% vital capacity?

5.   Respiration in Review:

    A.   Outline the process of normal quiet respiration:

    6.   A Brief Clinical Note: describe two ways disease can affect respiration for speech:

Section:

The Larynx and Phonation

Critical Concept:

The larynx is a protective structure located in the center of the neck. Formed of cartilage and muscle and covered by mucous membrane, it blocks the entry of foreign substances into the lower respiratory tract. It also provides most of the sound for speech by harnessing aerodynamic forces of exhalation in the process of phonation or voicing. Phonation is required for production of all vowels and for most consonants. In phonation, exhaled air acts on the twin true vocal folds when the tiny muscles of the larynx bring them into contact over the top of the trachea in concert with the muscles of respiration.

1. The Anatomy of the Larynx

    A.   Why does the chapter's author (Willard Zemlin) give the laryngeal cartilages the following nicknames?

        I. Ringlike Cricoid:

        ii. Shieldlike Thyroid:

        iii. Flexible Epiglottis:

        iv. Paired Arytenoids:

    B.   Which cartilage is attached to the first tracheal ring?

    C.   With which cartilage do the arytenoid cartilages articulate?

    D.   To which cartilages are the ends of the vocal ligaments attached?

E.   How does the articulation of the thyroid and cricoid cartilages change the tension of the vocal ligament?

F.   Which muscles act in opposition for cricothyroid rotation?

G.   What pair of muscles abducts the vocal ligaments?

H.   What are three factors that greatly influence the mode of vocal fold vibration? (*Hint: see the summary at the end of the "Laryngeal Physiology" section.*)

I.   Describe three ways disease can affect the vibration of the vocal folds:

       I.

       ii.

       iii.

2.   Laryngeal Physiology

   A.   What two forces account for the versatility of the voice?

   B.   What forces cause the vocal folds to vibrate?

   C.   What is the average frequency of vocal fold vibration in adults?

      I.   Males:

      ii.   Females:

   D.   Describe the events that take place during the following phases of the glottal cycle.

      I.   Opening Phase:

      ii.   Closing Phase:

      iii.   Closed Phase:

3.   The Pitch-Changing Mechanism

     A.   What is the relationship between pitch and the rate of glottal vibration?

     B.   Describe the forces that increase the frequency of the glottal vibration:

4.   The Loudness Mechanism

     A.   What change in the glottal cycle accompany increases in vocal loudness?

     B.   How does the respiratory system accommodate to increases in speech loudness?

Section:

Articulation

Critical Concept:

We may think of the upper respiratory tract as being in the shape of a resonating tube, running through the neck and skull, closed at the glottis and opened at the lips or nose. A speaker changes the cross sectional area of the tube to produce the vowels and sonorant consonants of speech and blocks the airflow with glottis, tongue or lip to create the turbulence of obstruent consonants.

1.   The Skeletal Framework of the Vocal Tract

     A.   What are the two major parts of the skull?

B.   What names have anatomists given to the first and second cervical vertebrae?

2.   Cavities and Associated Structures of the Vocal Tract

A.   Where is the *Buccal Cavity*?

B.   How does a speaker form constrictions along the vocal tract to produce obstruent consonants?

C.   What is the role of the muscles of facial expression in the production of speech?

3.   Dentition

A.   Describe the development of dentition from childhood until the twenties.

B.   How can the teeth contribute to facial growth?

4.   Tongue Musculature

   A.   What is the difference between *intrinsic* and *extrinsic* tongue musculature?

   B.   Describe the function of the *genioglossus* muscle. Is *genioglossus* an intrinsic or an extrinsic muscle?

   C.   In the space below, draw and label a diagram of the oral cavity. Use Figure 3.21 as a guide.

5.   Mandibular Movement

    A.   Describe three directions in which muscles move the mandible.

        I.

        ii.

        iii.

    B.   What speech sounds require the greatest mandibular elevation?

6.   The Soft Palate

    A.   Why does a speaker close off the nasal cavity when forming plosive sounds, like /p/ and /k/?

    B.   What the physical phenomenon we perceive as *nasality*?

    C.   Name the muscles that elevate the velum.

    D.   Name the muscles that depress the velum.

7.   The Pharynx

    A.   What are the main divisions of the pharynx?

    B.   Describe the contribution of the pharynx to speech articulation.

8   Articulatory Physiology

    A.   What are three dimensions in which the vocal tract may be altered for the purposes of speech

    B.   How do the lips affect speech articulation?

        I.   ...of consonants

        ii.   ...of vowels

9. Vowel Production

   A. What position does the tongue assume when a speaker uses the vowel /I/?

   B. What position does the tongue assume when a speaker uses the vowel /ɑ/?

   C. What is distinctive about the speech sounds we call *diphthongs*?

   D. Why do you think listeners tolerate more variation in vowel production than we do in consonant production?

10. Consonant Production

    A. Describe two differences between vowels and consonants.

       I.

       ii.

51

B. Review the *places* of consonant articulation. What oral structures does the speaker approximate when the target phonemes have the following places of articulation?

    I.   Bilabial:

    ii.   Labiodental:

    iii.   Dental:

    iv.   Alveolar:

    v.   Palatal:

    vi.   Velar:

    vii.   Glottal:

C. Describe the differences in manner of articulation between a *plosive* and a *fricative*.

D. What happens when the speaker produces an *affricate*?

E. How do semivowels function phonetically...

    I.   ...as consonants?

    ii.   ...as vowels?

F.   Identify the homophonous (voiced/voiceless) cognates for the plosives: /p/; /t/; and /k/ and the fricatives: /f/; /Ө/; /s/; and /ʃ/.

G.   Describe two abnormal conditions under which unwanted nasal resonance may affect speech.

   I.

   ii.

Section:

The Nervous System and Speech Production

Critical Concept:

All of our behavior is brought about through the interplay of input and output to and from the human nervous system. Whether conscious or unconscious, this interplay is the result of electrochemical changes in billions of neurons composing the central and peripheral divisions of the system. The seat of conscious thought, including language, is the brain. The neurons of brain activate lower level efferent neurons to contract the muscles of speech according to programmed patterns. In turn, lower level afferent neurons inform the brain about the accuracy of speech movements as they happen. One of the best ways to learn about the brain is to study how its parts form from three brain vesicles in the womb.

1. Neurons: In the box below, draw a diagram of a neuron. Use figure 3.30 as a guide. label the *cell body*; *axon*; and *dendrites*.

2. How are neurons like other cells in the body?

3. How are neurons different from other body cells?

4. Name the two major divisions of the human nervous system and describe their components.

5. What is the difference between an *afferent* neuron and an *efferent* neuron?

6.   **The Brain:**

    A.   Identify the adult brain structures that develop from the three primary vesicles of the infant's brain.

        i.   Forebrain:

        ii.   Midbrain:

        iii..   Hindbrain:

    B.   Identify the communication functions of the lobes of the cerebral cortex:

        I.   Frontal:

        ii.   Parietal:

        iii.   Temporal:

        iv.   Occipital:

C.   Describe the following nervous system disorders and identify which part of the forebrain may be damaged when each disorder occurs.

      I.   Athetosis:

      ii.   Ataxia:

      iii.   Ataxia:

      iv.   Nystagmus:

      v.   Aphasia:

D.   What is the *Thalamus*?

7.   Cranial Nerves: Using the diagram in figure 3.36 and accompanying text, name the twelve cranial nerves and briefly describe their functions in communication.

      I.

      II.

      III.

      IV.

      V.

VI.

VII.

VIII.

IX.

X.

XI.

XII.

8.   Where does the spinal cord begin and end?

9.   Name two differences between a cranial nerve and a spinal nerve:

Critical Terms

Define the following terms, using your text as a reference:

o   Larynx

o   Pharynx

o   Thorax

o   Tidal Volume

o   Residual Volume

o   Cricoid Cartilage

o   Vocal Tract

o   Glottis

o   Genioglossus

o   Velum

o   Axon

o   Cerebrum

o   Respiration

o   Oral Cavity

o   Trachea

o   Vital Capacity

o   Laryngeal Tone

o   Buccal Cavity

o   Mandible

- ○ Maxillae

- ○ Hard Palate

- ○ Diphthongs

- ○ Cognates

- ○ Dendrites

- ○ Brainstem

- ○ Respiratory Tract

- ○ Nasal Cavity

- ○ Alveoli

- ○ Bronchial Tubes

- ○ Hyoid Bone

- ○ Arytenoid Cartilage

- ○ Cranium

- ○ Cricothyroid Muscle

- ○ Thyroarytenoid Muscle

- ○ Neurons

- ○ CNS

- ○ Hindbrain

- ○ Phonation

- ○ Resonance

- ○ Diaphragm

- o Hyoid Bone

- o Thyroid Cartilage

- o PNS

- o Cerebral Cortex

Chapter Three Self Test

True/False

1. There is a wide a span of human anatomical attributes called "normal."
        True
        False
2. The larynx is built to withstand prolonged yelling.
        True
        False
3. We inhale by creating negative air pressure in the lungs:
        True
        False
4. Increased tension of in the vocal folds is usually accompanied by an increase in pitch.
        True
        False
5. The diaphragm is a muscle of exhalation.
        True
        False
6. The upper portion of the trunk is called the *abdomen*.
        True
        False
7. The vocal tract consists of the pharynx, oral cavity and nasal cavity.
        True
        False
8. Consonants are produced with a relatively open vocal tract.
        True
        False
9. The larynx excites the air in the upper respiratory tract.
        True
        False
10. Whispered vowels are always voiced.
        True
        False
11. The respiratory tract begins at the mouth and nose and ends deep in the lungs.
        True
        False
12. When we are not talking, we breathe quietly about twelve times each minute.
        True
        False

13.   The thorax contains the lungs.
        True
        False

14.   Most consonants require vibration of the vocal folds.
        True
        False

15.   The biomechanics of speech breathing are similar to those for vegetative breathing.
        True
        False

16.   Muscular force for exhalation is never required during speech.
        True
        False

17.   The diaphragm is a muscle of exhalation.
        True
        False

18.   We use our tidal respiratory volume during quiet breathing.
        True
        False

19.   The average vital capacity in adults ranges from 1000 to 1500 cc.
        True
        False

20.   The largest of the laryngeal cartilages is the thyroid cartilage.
        True
        False

21.   The permanent teeth are also known as the deciduous teeth.
        True
        False

22.   The cricothyroid muscle opposes the thyroarytenoid muscle.
        True
        False

23.   When the posterior cricoarytenoid muscles contract, the glottis becomes larger.
        True
        False

24.   The orbicularis oris muscle purses the lips.
        True
        False

25.   When the genioglossus muscle contracts, the tongue moves forward.
        True
        False

26.   The lower jaw is called the maxilla.
        True
        False

27. The pharynx is a dynamic articulator.
    True
    False
28. The velum is lowered for production of /m/.
    True
    False
29. A vowel produced with the tongue held high and forward will probably be recognized as /I/.
    True
    False
30. Voiced speech sounds are shaped by alterations in the configuration of the vocal tract.
    True
    False
31. The cranial nerves are located along the spinal cord.
    True
    False
32. The peripheral nervous system is contained in the skull and spinal column.
    True
    False
33. The temporal lobe is part of the forebrain.
    True
    False
34. Broca discovered that 90% of people who had damage to Broca's area on the left side also had aphasia.
    True
    False
35. We are born with an estimated 100 billion neurons.
    True
    False

Multiple Choice

1. The amount of air remaining in the lungs after a maximum exhalation is called:
    a. vital capacity
    b. functional reserve volume
    c. residual volume
    d. complemental air.
2. Which of the following is included among the human vocal organs?
    a. eyes
    b. ears
    c. larynx
    d. heart

3. A fairly regular series of air pulses is produced by the larynx during:
   a. phonation
   b. pronation
   c. phonetics
   d. phonics

4. An important role of hearing in normal speech is one of:
   a. reaction to danger
   b. maintenance of balance
   c. triggering the stapedial reflex
   d. providing feedback

5. During the speech act, the muscles of muscles of inhalation perform which function?
   a. partially defeat excessive relaxation pressure
   b. produce micro-movements for phonation
   c. draw air into the lungs
   d. increase airflow rate during utterance of stressed syllables

6. Neurogenic respiratory disorders may result in:
   a. lack of control of inhalation
   b. inability to switch from vegetative to speech breathing
   c. inappropriate active exhalation
   d. all of the above

7. The muscle thought to be primarily responsible for shortening and opposing tension on the vocal folds is the:
   a. posterior cricoarytenoid
   b. lateral cricoarytenoid
   c. cricothyroid
   d. thyroarytenoid

8. The laryngeal cartilage shaped like a ring is the:
   a. cricoid
   b. epiglottis
   c. arytenoid
   d. thyroid

9. The vocal ligaments attach to which part of each arytenoid cartilage?
   a. muscular process
   b. vocal process
   c. cricothyroid process
   d. apex

10. The function of the posterior cricoarytenoid muscles is to:
    a. adduct the vocal ligaments
    b. abduct the vocal ligaments
    c. increase tension on the vocal ligaments
    d. decrease tension in the vocal ligaments

11. A muscle important in increasing tension of the vocal folds is the:
    a. posterior cricoarytenoid
    b. lateral cricoarytenoid
    c. thyroarytenoid
    d. cricothyroid
12. Adult female vocal folds vibrate at about:
    a. 65 times per second
    b. 10,000 times per second
    c. 120-145 times per second
    d. 200-260 times per second
13. The *Rima Glottidis* is:
    a. the pharynx
    b. the space between the teeth and the cheeks
    d. the space between the true margins of the vocal folds
    e. the oral cavity
14. Which of the following may affect the sound of the voice?:
    a. medial compression, longitudinal tension and subglottic pressure
    b. smoking alcohol and polluted air
    c. mass changes caused by inflammation of the vocal folds
    d. all of the above
15. The functional cells of the nervous system are called :
    a. glial cells
    b. neurons
    c. oligodendroglia
    d. end brushes
16. Raised areas on the surface of the cerebrum are called:
    a. nuclei
    b. gyri
    c. sulci
    d. ventricles
17. Speech is what kind of respiratory function??
    a. digestive
    b. circulatory
    c. respiratory
    d. biosocial
18. In which part of the brain are the cranial nerve nuclei located?
    a. forebrain and basal ganglia
    b. midbrain and hindbrain
    c. cerebellum
    d. corpus callosum

19. The vocal tract behaves acoustically like a:
    a. a tube, closed at one end and open at the other
    b. a box with no top
    c. a pair of strings, anchored at both ends
    d. a reed
20. The resonances of the vocal tract are called:
    a. fundamentals
    b. formants
    c. overtones
    d. volume
21. On which vertebra does the skull rest?:
    a. Vertebra Prominens
    b. Atlas
    c. Axis
    d. T-12
22. Deciduous teeth are commonly called:
    a. permanent teeth
    b. "baby teeth"
    c. front teeth
    d. molars
23. The roof of the oral cavity is formed by parts of the .
    a. mandible
    b. maxilla
    c. velum
    d. thyroid
24. The nasal and pharyngeal cavities are coupled through action of the:
    a. maxilla
    b. epiglottis
    c. velum
    d. all of the above
25. The opening between the true margins of the vocal folds is called the:
    a. epiglottis
    b. glottis
    c. pharynx
    d. none of the above
26. Approximation of the vocal folds is called:
    a. medial compression
    b. longitudinal tension
    c. phonation
    d. subglottal air pressure

27. The three divisions of the pharynx are:
    a. vestibule, ventricle and subglottic area
    b. nasopharynx, oropharynx and laryngopharynx
    c. labiopharynx, linguopharynx and glottidopharynx
    d. frontal, parietal and occipital

28. Cognate pairs differ in terms of which feature?
    a. manner of articulation
    b. tongue placement
    c. presence or absence of phonation
    d. tongue height

29. The muscle that protrudes the tongue is called:
    a. palatoglossus
    b. hyoglossus
    c. genioglossus
    d. linguoglossus

30. The muscles that move the mandible can be grouped functionally into:
    a. elevators
    b. depressors
    c. a protractor
    d. all of the above

31. The articulators change the shape (and acoustic characteristics) of the vocal tract in which of the following dimensions?
    a. overall length
    b. location of constriction
    c. degree of constriction
    d. all of the above

32. The vowel /u/ may be described as:
    a. close front
    b. close back
    c. open front
    d. open back

33. A blend of two separate vowels may be called a:
    a. close front vowel
    b. monophthong
    c. diphthong
    d. triphthong

34. The places of consonant articulation include:
    a. mandibular
    b. labiodental
    c. cranial
    d. orbicular

35. Sounds generated with rapid articulatory movement, and without prominent noise or turbulence are called:
        a. diphthongs
        b. affricates
        c. homophones
        d. glides

> # Chapter Four Students' Guide
>
> ## Communication Differences and Disorders
>
> Kay T. Payne and Orlando L. Taylor

Chapter Summary

Speech-language pathologists appreciate that language cognition and culture are inseparably bound. According to the author, the four most populous cultural groups in the United States are Native American, African American, Hispanic American and Asian American. There are many more cultural groups, and each may have its own style, language and pragmatic aspects in interpersonal communication. Accurate evaluation of a person's communicative abilities must distinguish between a communicative difference and a communicative disorder.

Student Outcomes

After reading this chapter students should be able to do the following:

☞ Contrast LANGUAGE DISORDER and LANGUAGE DIFFERENCE.

☞ Describe the relationship between LANGUAGE and CULTURE and major factors which influence language behavior.

☞ Describe the concept of dialectical variation.

☞ Describe the influence of other languages on English.

☞ Discuss social reactions to DIALECTICAL DIFFERENCES.

☞ Discuss the role of the Speech-Language Pathologists in addressing dialectical and language differences.

☞ Contrast the concepts of BILINGUAL and BIDIALECTICAL.

☞ Describe cultural bias in assessment and intervention for speakers who do not speak what is considered to be standard English.

Critical Concepts

Section

Basic Concepts Related to Culture and Language

Concept

Since the language of a cultural group reflects that group's motivations, ideas and beliefs, that language will be strongly flavored by the culture. Culture is distinct from race, nationality, religion, language or socioeconomic status.

1. How is culture different from *race*?.

2. Saville-Trioke (1978) claimed that culture tends to be characterized by conduct in twenty areas. Describe how members of your culture behave in the following areas. (*Suggestion: compare your responses with those of friends or class members from various cultural groups).*

    A.   Family Structure:

    B.   Important Events in Life Cycle:

    C.   Roles of Individual Members:

D.   Rules of Interpersonal Interactions:

E.   Communication and Linguistic Rules:

F.   Rules for Decorum and Discipline:

G.   Religious Beliefs:

H.   Standards for Health and Hygiene:

I.   Food Preferences:

J.   Dress and Personal Appearance:

K.   History and Traditions:

L.   Holidays and Celebrations:

M.   Value and Methods:

N.   Education:

O.   Perceptions of Work and Play:

P.   Perceptions of Time and Space:

Q.   Explanation of Natural Phenomena:

R.   Attitudes Towards Pets and Animals:

S.   Artistic and Musical Values and Taste:

T.   Life Expectations and Aspirations:

2.   How does *sociolinguistics* contribute to the field of speech-language pathology?

3.   Differentiate between a *language dialect* and an *accent*. What is *code switching*?

4.   How does *ethnicity* influence communicative behavior?

5.   Describe how *social class, education* and *occupation* influence communicative behavior in the following areas.

A.   Home Environment:

B.   Child Rearing Practices:

C.   Access to Other Cultures:

6.   Name seven regional (stereotyped) dialects of English seen in the United States.

7.   What are five determinants of regional dialect according to Wardhaugh (1976)?

8.   Describe five linguistic gender differences observed in the United States.

9.   How might *situation* affect language use during a speech-language evaluation?

10.   How does *peer group association* affect your own language use?

11.   Describe three ways that early experiences may affect later language learning.

Section:

Dialects of American English

Concept:

Historically, English has been influenced by other languages, and American English is no exception. Since the demographic makeup of the United States is so diverse, the influences on American English are many.

1.   Describe how the following seven factors caused dialectical variation in American English.

    A.   Importation of language features by various cultural groups:

    B.   Influence of indigenous language:

    C.   Mixing of adjacent cultural communities:

    D.   Power:

    E.   Migration within the country:

    F.   Geographic isolation:

    G.   Self-imposed social isolation:

2.   What group speaks *African American English*.

3.   What is the *creolist* theory of African American English evolution?

4.   State two arguments against the creolist theory.

5.   What is a *pidgin* language?

6.   What is the difference between language *influence* and language *interference*?

7.   In general, describe how your own culture manages the following pragmatic communicative acts.

        A.   Opening or Closing a Conversation:

        B.   Turn-taking During Conversations:

C.   Interruptions:

D.   Silence as a Communicative Device:

E.   Appropriate Topics of Conversation:

F.   Humor and When to Use It:

G.   Nonverbal Modes to Accompany Conversation:

H.   Laughter as a Communicative Device:

I.   Appropriate Amount of Speech to Be Used by Participants:

J.   Logical Ordering of Events Used During Discourse:

8.   What is the difference between *oral* strategies and *literate* strategies in narration?

9.   Describe the four characteristics of a *topic centered* narrative.

10.   How does personal health affect communication?

Section:

Language Differences and Communication Disorders

Concept:

Speech-language pathologists and audiologists regard communication as a widely variable behavior, and view individual and cultural differences as an inherent quality of humanity. If a client is to gain from the services of the communication professional, her or his linguistic function must be assessed and treated within the context of individual needs and cultural standards.

1.   How do a society's attitudes about communication and language determine when a language *difference* is a *disorder* and what constitutes its best treatment?

2.   Describe how standardized tests may be biased in Taylor's (1978; 1983) seven dimensions.

   A.   Social Situational Bias:

   B.   Value Bias:

   C.   Phonological Bias:

   D.   Grammatical Bias:

E.   Vocabulary Bias:

F.   Pragmatic Bias:

G.   Directions/Format Bias:

3.   How do "whites" differ from African Americans in stuttering behavior according to Leith and Mims (1975)?

4.   What is the major consideration in assessing language development in a child who is a speaker of a non-standard dialect?

5.   List five possible steps (Feigenbaum, 1970) in the process of teaching standard English to speakers of non-standard dialects and show how Taylor's (1986) eight steps correspond to them.

                 Feigenbaum   Taylor

        A.

        B.

C.

D.

E.

Critical Terms

Define the following terms, using your text as a reference:

o   Accent

o   Dialect

o   Culture

o   Sociolinguistics

o   Domain

o   Vernacular

o   Ethnography of Communication

o   Bilingual

o   Bidialectical

o   Motherese

o   Code-Switching

o   Black English

o   Pidgin

o   Creolist Theory

o   Decreolization

o   Narratives

o   Oral Strategies

o   Literate Strategies

o   Topic Centered Narratives

o   Topic Associated Narratives

Chapter Four Self Test

True/False

1. Cultural groups may vary in several aspects of language use.
    True
    False
2. Dialects of a language include deep structure as well as surface structure.
    True
    False
3. The terms *regional dialects* and *accent* have the same meaning.
    True
    False
4. Dialects and accents are language disorders.
    True
    False
5. If a dialect results in ridicule of the speaker, it is a communication disorder.
    True
    False
6. Culture is learned.
    True
    False
7. Standardized language proficiency tests are relatively valid if the cultural background of the person being tested is represented in the test's standardization sample.
    True
    False
8. Culture may be represented by standards for health and hygiene.
    True
    False
9. Members of the same race may have different cultures.
    True
    False
10. Dialects of social groups are easily changed by outside forces.
    True
    False
11. Ethnic influences on language are basically biological in nature.
    True
    False
12. Individuals may speak several dialects.
    True
    False

13. Membership in a cultural group is a good predictor of language form.
    True
    False

14. Inhabitants of a geographic region belong to the same speech community.
    True
    False

15. Child rearing styles may affect meal length of utterance in children.
    True
    False

16. The Creolist Theory is currently accepted by all sociolinguists.
    True
    False

17. Sociolinguists recognize three regional dialects in the continental United States.
    True
    False

18. Some phonological characteristics of Southern White Nonstandard English are also characteristic of African American English .
    True
    False

19. Gender is not related to language use.
    True
    False

20. Code-switching enables a speaker to use more than one language or dialect.
    True
    False

21. Situation or context may have an effect on language use.
    True
    False

22. Standard English is "White" English.
    True
    False

23. Bilingual speakers may code switch as a situation demands.
    True
    False

24. African American phonology may substitute voiceless labiodental fricatives where voiceless interdental fricatives occur in the standard dialect.
    True
    False

25. Culture has no discernable effect on stuttering characteristics
    True
    False

26. According to ASHA policy, accent reduction is outside the scope of practice of speech-language pathologists.

                True

                False

Multiple Choice

1. The Creole theory suggests that African American English derived from which of the following languages?
    a. Dutch
    b. French
    c. English
    d. all of the above and more

2. Which of the following is not a component of *accent*:
    a. semantics
    b. phonology
    c. suprasegmental characteristics
    d. vocal characteristics

3. Individuals who speak two languages are said to be:
    a. biglossal.
    b. bicyclical.
    c. bidialectical.
    d. bilingual

4. Variations within a language that include deep structure and linguistic codes are termed:
    a. dialects
    b. accents
    c. vernaculars
    d. narratives

5. Which of the following influences language and communication?
    a. ethnicity
    b. social class
    c. gender
    d. all of the above

6. Which of the following is a regional dialect?
    a. Creole
    b. African American
    c. Asian American
    d. Southern American

7. Which of the following speech differences have investigators associated with gender?
    a. mean length of utterance
    b. type-token ratio
    c. joking
    d. lying

8. According to the author, which of the following distinguishes Standard (American) English from its dialectical variants?
    a. deep structure
    b. use of pronouns
    c. linguistic and structural characteristics
    d. vocal patterns, phrase and word and phrase emphases

9. Research has shown that simultaneous acquisition of two languages may occur without negative interaction prior to what age?:
    a. 21 years
    b. 3 years
    c. 12 years
    d. 30 years

10. African American English s the linguistic code used by:
    a. Africans
    b. all African Americans
    c. Southern Americans
    d. working-class African Americans

11. The majority of African American utterances conform to the rules of
    a. Creole English
    b. Appalachian English
    c. Southern American English
    d. General American English

12. Who is among a small group of scholars who account for the full range of language use by African American people in the United States?
    a. K. Payne
    b. O. Taylor
    c. W. Secord
    d. E. Wiig

13. The largest group of in the United States today with native language influence on English consists of people from which background?
    a. French
    b. Hebrew
    c. Scottish
    d. Spanish

14. Oral-based cultures value:
    a. literature
    b. poetry
    c. speech
    d. all of the above

15. Which of the following type of stories is used by working-class children?
    a. topic associated
    b. standardized
    c. fairy tales
    d. historical

16. Most of the standardized tests used by speech-language pathologists are based on which variant of American English?
    a. Northern Midland
    b. New York
    c. Southwestern
    d. African American

17. Mismatch between the rules of communication interaction between the test maker and the test taker may be termed:
    a. social/situational bias
    b. phonological bias
    c. pragmatic bias
    d. format bias

18. Which of the following is a good solution to standardized test bias?
    a. Never use standardize tests in an evaluation.
    b. Develop criterion-references tests.
    c. Publish African American versions of all standardized tests.
    d. Limit evaluation sessions to thirty minutes.

19. "I might could'a done it," is an example of a:
    a. relative clause
    b. intensifying adverb
    c. consonant cluster reduction
    d. double modal

20. Age, education, and situation typically influence:
    a. code-switching efficacy are
    b. gender, race, and socioeconomic status
    c. region, intelligence, and personality
    d. none of the above.

21. The "Ann Arbor Decision" (1977) outlawed which of the following?
    a. use of dialect in public schools
    b. failure to place culturally different children in speech therapy
    c. inappropriate placement in treatment based on language differences
    d. use of standardized tests

22. Which of the following is a characteristic of men's language?
    a. precise articulation
    b. apologizing
    c. profanity in formal mixed company
    d. avoiding confrontation

Chapter Five Students' Guide

Language Disorders in Preschool Children

Amy M. Wetherby

Chapter Summary

Chapter five presents a comprehensive view of language disorders in very young children. Reflecting the author's deep personal and professional involvement in the field, it includes a wide array of information regarding classification and causes of language impairment. The chapter completes the picture by presenting variations in approaches to case management for children with language disorders and emphasizes the importance of home treatment support from their families or caregivers.

Student Outcomes

After reading and lecture, the students will:

☞ Apply constructivist and transactional perspectives to the roles of the child and the caregiver in management of communicative disorders.

☞ Discuss limitations of the traditional medical diagnostic classification systems in management of communication disorders in very young children.

☞ Contrast causes of primary and secondary language disorders.

☞ Apply the components of the Individualized Family Service Plan to the treatment of a child with a primary and one secondary language disorder.

☞ Apply the components of the Individualized Family Service Plan to the treatment of a child with a secondary language disorder.

☞ Describe three advantages each of norm-referenced measurement, criterion-referenced measurement and performance assessment in their applications to evaluation and assessment of communication disorders.

☞ Apply the principles of curricular planning, activity planning and scaffolding to enhancing content and context in whole language stimulation.

☞ Apply the principles of direct teaching, incidental teaching and milieu intervention to center-based and home-based management of preschool communication disorders.

Critical Concepts

Section:

Nature of Language Disorders in Young Children

Concept:

The first major section of this chapter describes the causes and effects of communication disorders in children. These disorders of communication are among the most common and pervasive disabilities of early childhood, affecting about 10-15 % of school-aged children. The section begins with a brief review of the evolution of educators' and others' approaches to language from a collection of rules to learn to a developmental process based on interactions with other language users in the environment. Several diseases and conditions may affect the interactions between a child and the environment, including specific language impairment, mental disabilities, pervasive developmental disorders, traumatic brain injury and environmental deprivation.

1. Developmental Framework.

    A. Describe the following approaches language development:

        i. Constructivist perspective.

        ii. Transactional perspective.

B.   How might a switch from a constructivist to a transactional approach to language development affect service delivery in speech-language pathology?

2.   How might factors in a caregiver affect a child's transactional language development?

3.   How might factors in a child affect developmental transactions?

Section:

Nature of Language Problem-Form, Content, Use

Concept:

Children with language disorders have impairments in their abilities to receive, process and transmit the symbols of language. Language disorders have been classified under several medical systems, but these models have limitations when dealing with such a complex aspect of human developmental behavior.

1.   In the space below, describe the difference between primary and secondary language disorders. Give two examples of each.

2.   Under which section of DSM IV are communication disorders in children placed?

3.   Describe the limitations of a medical diagnostic model for childhood language disorders/

Section:

Causal Factors

Concept:

Causes of language disorders may be traced to conditions inherent in the individual's constitution present before, during, or after birth. A poor language learning environment may be the basis for language delay alone or may interact with biological factors to worsen the problem.

1.   Describe the difference between environmental and biological risk factors for communicative disorders.

2.   Name two biological congenital conditions that might affect language development occurring at each of the following stages.

   A.   Prenatal

   B.   Perinatal

   C.   Postnatal

3.   Name three environmental conditions that may affect language development.

   A.

   B.

   C.

4.   How are language disorders related to academic performance?

5.   How are language disorders related to emotional adjustment?

Section:

Children with Specific Receptive-/Expressive Language Disorders

Concept:

When a child has a disorder affecting language independent of other neurological functions, the disorder is termed "Specific Language Impairment," or "SLI." SLI is characterized by late and restricted development of symbolic skills, including word, concept, and grammar knowledge, but normal non-verbal performance.

1.   At what age are most cases of specific language impairment identified?

2.   What is the relationship between vocabulary development and language disability?

3.   What are typical developmental trends in syntactic and discourse development among children with specific language impairment?

Section:

Children with Mental Disabilities

Concept:

Children with mental disabilities (mental retardation) function below the levels of most children their ages on intellectual and adaptive measures. Most, but not all, have language comprehension and production levels commensurate with their cognitive levels. Mental disabilities can be biological or environmental in origin.

1.   What is an *Intelligence Quotient*?

2.   Give the I.Q. ranges for mental disabilities of the following extents:

   A.   Mild:

   B.   Moderate:

   C.   Severe:

   D.   Profound:

3.   What are the limitations of I.Q. measurement with very young children?

Section:

Children with Autism and Pervasive Developmental Disorder

Concept:

Pervasive Developmental Disorders (PDD) are aberrations in childhood behavior that are characterized by impaired social interaction, impairment in verbal and nonverbal behavior and insistence on sameness. Some children manifest only some of these features. The cause is unknown, but appears to be neurogenic.

1.   Describe the following characteristics of pervasive developmental disorders.

    A.   Impaired social interaction:

    B.   Verbal and nonverbal behavior impairment:

    C.   Insistence on sameness:

2.   Describe the following communicative characteristics of children with pervasive developmental disorder.

    A.   Verbal or nonverbal?

    B.   Pragmatic skills:

    C.   Echolalia:

Section:

Children with Traumatic Brain Injury

Concept:

Children who suffer traumatic brain injury as a result of accident or abuse demonstrate behavioral traits different than those of brain injured adults. Prognosis depends upon the age at which a child was injured, since cerebral functions are most plastic before age two.

1.   Is brain injury in children more likely to be diffuse or focal?

2.   What is the most common cause of death in abused infants?

3.   In what ways are the results of brain injury in children different than those in adults? Describe how those differences change after two years of age.

4.   What is special about the left cerebral hemisphere?

Section:

Children At-Risk Due to Environmental Factors

Concept:

Research has suggested that language delays are among several of the dramatic detriments of impoverished environments. The benefits of language rich and verbally encouraging environments may begin at birth, making the preschool years of crucial importance.

1.   What two environmental elements are essential for language development?

2.   What three major differences did Hart and Risley (1994) find among 42 families?

       A.

       B.

       C.

3.   What two variables did Hart and Risley (1994) identify in the language parents used with their children?

4.   What did Hart and Risley (1994) conclude?

Section:

Service Delivery Models for Infants, Toddlers and Preschool Children

Concept:

Individual family service plans (IFSP's) are mandated by federal law to establish special educational intervention for preschool children years in home-based or center-based programs. Each IFSP is designed for the individual child and is implemented by a team consisting of appropriate professionals and emphasizing participation of family members.

1.   Briefly state the mandates of the following acts of congress:

        A.   Public law 94-142

        B.   Public law 99-457 part B

        C.   Public law 99-457 part H

2.   How did congress encourage compliance with these acts?

3. Why are there both *home-based* and *center-based* programs?

4. What does the author mean when she differentiates *child-centered* from *discipline-centered?*

Section:

Assessment Issues and Strategies

Concept:

There are two purposes for evaluation and assessment of communication abilities in young children. The first purpose is to establish whether a communicative disorder exists. The second purpose is to distinguish a disorder from others which may have similar symptoms. Identification of the disorder is augmented with evaluation and assessment of children's knowledge, abilities and achievements to provide information and guidelines about intervention planning.

1. Distinguish between screening, evaluation and assessment.

2. What is *eligibility* and why is it important to verify it?

Section:

Norm-Referenced Measures

Concept:

Norm-referenced measurement offers comparisons of the performance of a particular child with those of normal groups and is important for establishing placement eligibility. Evaluators who employ norm-referenced instruments are trained to be familiar with their psychometric validity, reliability and contextual limitations.

1.   Why are the following characteristics of a norm-referenced instrument's standardization sample important for an examiner to consider when testing a particular child?

A.   Size

B.   Geographic origins

C.   Socioeconomic status of their families

D.   Ethnicity

E.   Health

2.   How is receptive language usually measured by norm-referenced instruments?

3.   How is expressive language usually measured by norm-referenced instruments

4.   Why is *reliability* important in a norm-referenced instrument?

5.   Why is *validity* important in a norm-referenced instrument?

Section:

Criterion-Referenced Measures

Concept:

Formal and informal criterion-referenced measurement allows the child to demonstrate competence in a particular set of tasks. It is most useful for intervention planning.

1.   Why is criterion-referenced assessment most useful for intervention planning?

2.   What is the difference between a *formal* criterion-referenced device and an *informal* one?

Section:

Limitations of Assessment Tools for Young Children

Concept:

Current assessment procedures are limited in the content and scope of the information they gather as well as in the means by which they gather it.

1. Name four limitations of current assessment instruments.

    A.

    B.

    C.

    D.

2. How would you design an instrument to address these limitations?

    A.

    B.

    C.

    D.

Section:

Performance Assessment

Concept:

Performance assessment is controlled sampling of children's language and behavior in a variety of contexts. Clinicians individualize assessment contexts to meet the needs of the individual child and family.

1.   In what way does performance assessment address the limitations of other assessment means?

2.   What are the shortcomings of performance assessment?

Section:

Assessment for Identification

Concept:

Often the first evidence that a child has a developmental problem is delayed speech onset. Since delayed speech is not usually evident until the second year, this leads to delay in identification of very young children who need speech or language services. Clinicians must observe preverbal communication behavior which utilizes vocal and gestural modalities and indicates the ability to pretend in play to maximize the impact of the language environment during the first two years of life.

1. What is the rationale for assessment in children younger than two years? Should all children receive such an assessment?

2. List six early intervention indicators reported by Paul (1991) and Wetherby & Prizant (1993).

    A.

    B.

    C.

    D.

    E.

    F.

Section:

Assessment for Program Planning

Concept:

Once the clinician establishes placement eligibility through norm-referenced evaluation, criterion-referenced and performance based assessment strategies are most valuable for planning intervention strategies. Effective planning is enhanced by gathering information from a variety of sources, particularly in collaboration with family members.

1. What information might a clinician gain by observing a child's behavior in the presence of a caregiver?

2. What information might family members provide?

3. What information might direct observation provide?

4. Name three specific areas you might wish to observe as an assessing clinician.

    A.

    B.

    C.

Section:

Intervention Approaches and Strategies

Concept:

Developments in therapeutic paradigms offer more effective language learning contexts in comparison to the familiar "pull-out" treatment approach.

Section:

Content and Context of Language Intervention

Concept:

The goal of language intervention is to make the child a more effective communicator and learner. Clinicians base treatment activities on children's present language capacities in three contextual tiers that address the leaning environment.

1.   What is "inclusive" about "inclusive education"?

2.   What is the ultimate goal of language intervention?

3.   What treatment emphasis is appropriate for children with emerging language?

4.   What treatment emphasis is appropriate for children with emerging discourse?

5.   What are the three tiers of program planning?

        A.

        B.

        C.

6.   What does the author mean by chid-directed, as opposed to teacher-directed, special education?

7.   How can a child's family contribute to theme building in curriculum planning?

8.   Why do you think the *whole language* approach holds it important to include all language modalities in preschool education curriculum planning?

9.   List three advantages of a whole language approach.

     A.

     B.

     C.

10.   List two benefits of predictability and structure in curricular activities:

     A.

     B.

Section:

Specific Language Intervention Techniques

Concept:

Several teaching techniques may enhance the time tested direct technique for language stimulation. Incidental teaching and milieu intervention allow the child to direct the attention focus with the support of an adult.

1.   Develop an imaginary lesson during with the goal of teaching children how to perform a daily function, such as setting the table or dressing with the direct teaching, the incidental teaching and the milieu intervention technique. (*Use a separate sheet).*

2.   Which intervention strategy do you think the author of this chapter advocates the most? Which do you think she advocates the least?

13.   Which strategy does the author report is supported by empirical findings?

Section:

Collaboration with Families

Concept:

Public law has recognized that the family, not the professional, is constant the child's life. Five principles of family-centered practice provide guidelines for the family service professionals who work with family members to facilitate home language environment enrichment.

1.   List the five principles of family-centered practice (Dunst, Trivette, Starnes, Hanby and Gordon, 1993) and describe why each one is important.

A.

B.

C.

D.

E.

2.	How would you apply these principles in helping a family manage a child with communication problems?

Critical Terms

Define the following terms, using your text as a reference:

o   Constructivist Perspective

o   Transactional Perspective

o   Pragmatics

o   Primary Language Disorder

o   Secondary Language Disorder

o   DSM IV

o   Language Form

o   Language Content

o   Language Use

o   Failure to Thrive

o   Specific Language Impairment

o   Late Bloomers

o   Late Talkers

o   Pervasive Developmental Disorders

o   Traumatic Brain Injury

o   Public Laws: 94-142; 99-457

o   Individual Educational Program

o   Individual Family Service Plan

o   Home-Based Program

o   Center-Based Program

o   Evaluation

o   Assessment

o   Norm-Referenced Measures

o   Reliability

o   Validity

o   Criterion-Referenced Measures

o   Performance Assessment

o   Language Context

o   Inclusive Education

o   Emerging Literacy

o   Emerging Discourse

o   Curricular Planning

o   Activity Planning

o   Scaffolding

o   Joint Action Routine

o   Direct Teaching

o   Incidental Teaching

o   Milieu Intervention

o   Modeling

o   Mand-Model Procedure

Chapter Five Self Test

True/False

1. About 75% of school children have speech, language or hearing disorders.
    True
    False

2. The semantic revolution was rooted in the cognitive theories of Piaget.
    True
    False

3. Standardized language tests are useful for making decisions about eligibility.
    True
    False

4. The pragmatic approach to language function emphasizes the social utility of language.
    True
    False

5. Language development is independent of contextual considerations.
    True
    False

6. The psychological well-being of the caregiver has little or no influence on a child's successful language acquisition.
    True
    False

7. A secondary language disorder is presumed to be caused by biological factors.
    True
    False

8. Cerebral palsy is an example of a biological risk factor for language disorders.
    True
    False

9. Child maltreatment can include failure of caregivers to produce a stimulating environment.
    True
    False

10. The severity of a communication disorder cannot be easily predicted from known risk factors.
    True
    False

11. Discourse is the ability to connect one sentence to another.
    True
    False

12. The effects of brain injury on an infant brain may be reliably inferred from observations of similar injuries on adult brains.
    True
    False

13. A child with a measured IQ in the range of 50-70 is considered mentally disabled.
    True
    False

14. Mental disability is diagnosed according to intellect and adaptation skills.
    True
    False

15. Echolalia may be a language learning strategy for children with pervasive developmental disorders.
    True
    False

16. Both cerebral hemispheres have the capacity to learn language.
    True
    False

17. Early intervention programs for children with language delays should begin before age four.
    True
    False

18. Federal law provides financial incentives for developing language stimulation programs for infants and toddlers.
    True
    False

19. Hart and Risley (1995) found no difference in home stimulation associated with socioeconomic status.
    True
    False

20. Federal regulations require establishment of an Individualized Family Service Plan
    True
    False

21. Assessment refers to the process used to determine a child's eligibility for treatment services.
    True
    False

22. Criterion-referenced measures measure a child's level of performance in a specific domain.
    True
    False

23. Early assessment tools are limited in scope.
        True
        False
24. Inclusive treatment programs limit opportunities for typical peer interaction.
        True
        False
25. Whole language approaches integrate all language modalities.
        True
        False
26. The ultimate goal of language intervention is to make the child a more effective communicator and learner.
        True
        False
27. Inclusive education is mandated by public law.
        True
        False
28. Children benefit from predictability and structure.
        True
        False
29. Drawing is an early form of writing.
        True
        False
30. Current research supports milieu intervention as the best language teaching approach.
        True
        False

Multiple Choice:

1. The perspective of language development that emphasizes role of language in ordering a child's environment is the
    a. the grammatical approach.
    b. the transactional approach.
    c. the constructivist approach.
    d. the interpretive approach.
2. A primary language impairment may be caused by:
    a. visual impairment.
    b. orofacial paralysis.
    c. mental retardation.
    d. none of the above.

3. The most widely used diagnostic system in the medical profession is:
    a. Diagnostic and Statistical manual of Mental Disorders: IV.
    b. Merck's Manual.
    c. Burros Mental Measurements Yearbook.
    d. Manual of Medical Professions.
4. The most notable language characteristics of children with SLI include...
    a. echolalia.
    b. adolescent onset.
    c. semantic and grammatical deficits.
    d. intellectual and adaptive delays.
5. One of the best determinants of a child's outcome is...
    a. age of onset.
    b. the combined number of risk factors.
    c. maternal health.
    d. socioeconomic status of the family.
6. For children under age three, which is better used for assessment of mental disabilities?
    a. measure of developmental functioning
    b. a standardized intelligence test
    c. parent questionnaire
    d. all of the above
7. Intelligence quotients below 20 are classified as:
    a. mildly retarded
    b. moderately retarded
    c. severely retarded
    d. profoundly retarded
8. In children with PDD, what may pronoun reversal signify?
    a. rejection of the caregiver
    b. mental retardation
    c. use of language learning strategy
    d. sensory deficits
7. Swelling and edema following brain injury can lead to:
    a. generalized symptoms
    b. focal deficits
    c. specific language impairment
    d. Broca's aphasia
8. Special educational programs in the schools are documented which form?
    a. Health Care Finance Administration form #700
    b. Individual Family Service Plan
    c. Individual Educational Program
    d. clinical progress notes

9. The process of determining a child's eligibility for services includes:
    a. standardized test scores
    b. assessment protocols
    c. curriculum planning
    d. plan of treatment

10. Ongoing procedures used to identify the child's strengths and needs are part of which process?
    a. assessment
    b. evaluation
    c. I.Q. testing
    d. achievement testing

11. An intelligence quotient is usually inferred from which type of measurement?
    a. performance assessment
    b. criterion referenced testing
    c. informal assessment
    d. norm referenced testing

12. Validity of parental reports are greatly enhanced under which circumstances?
    a. The parents are allowed to report as a team.
    b. Parents have high socioeconomic status.
    c. Parents are given an inventory and focus on current skills.
    d. Parents are interviewed separately.

13. The normal age for emerging discourse is:
    a. 6 months
    b. 12 months
    c. 18 months
    d. 24 months

14. What is the role of the teacher in curricular planning?
    a. establish eligibility for speech therapy
    b. establish treatment goals and objectives
    c. prepare the learning environment and plan experiences
    d. supervise the speech-language pathologist

15. Using themes to enhance concept development is called what?
    a. theme building
    b. whole language approach
    c. direct teaching
    d. pull-out therapy

16. What is probably the most important time to begin inclusion?
    a. infancy
    b. early childhood
    c. adolescence
    d. There is never a good time to begin inclusion.

17. Which modality is emphasized in a whole language approach?
    a. spoken language
    b. written language
    c. gestural language
    d. all of the above

18. In language stimulation, what does "JAR" mean?
    a. joined activity regulation
    b. joint action routine
    c. Treatment objectives are written down and placed in a small glass container.
    d. Treatment results come as a surprise to the clinician and the child.

19. Typical and atypical children learn in the same classroom in which model?
    a. segregative model
    b. integrative model
    c. joint action routine
    d inclusive model

20. Through which teaching method does the teacher systematically present stimuli, elicit an expected response and provide consistent consequences?
    a. direct teaching
    b. inclusion
    c. incidental teaching
    d. milieu intervention

21. What does scaffolding provide for a child learning language?
    a. grammar
    b. contextual support
    c. incidental teaching
    d. success

22. Literacy begins at which developmental stage?
    a. infancy
    b. early childhood
    c. elementary school age
    d. adolescence

23. Which teaching technique has been established as superior?
    a. direct teaching
    b. indirect teaching
    c. milieu intervention
    d. none of the above

24. Which public law mandates family centered practice?
    a. 94-142
    b. 99-457
    c. IDEA
    d. 101-457

25. Which of the following are part of the grieving process?
    a. denial
    b. anxiety
    c. guilt
    d. all of the above.

Chapter Six Students' Guide

Language Disabilities in School-Age Children and Youth

Elisabeth H. Wiig and Wayne A. Secord

Chapter Summary

Language disabilities in school aged children interfere with their abilities to receive the full benefits of education during the critical years. Language-learning disabilities may affect all aspects of language, including word association abilities and pragmatic abilities. Attention Deficit Disorders (ADD) and Attention Deficit Hyperactivity Disorders (ADHD) m interfere with a student's ability to attend to instruction. These disabilities are neurogenic, and may result from injury or have genetic origins. special strategies appear effective in helping the person with language disability cope with the disorder, but treatment depends upon adequate evaluation and ongoing assessment. Since language function enhances a person's cognitive interaction with the world, language disorders are often accomapanied by personality adjustment problems. In such cases, effective treatment indicates counseling in addition to language treatment.

Student Outcomes

After reading this chapter, students should be able to do the following:

☞   Describe the major characteristics and causes of learning disabilities.

☞   Discuss the advantages of a multiple-strategy approach in the assesment of learning disabilities.

☞   Distinguish the possible effects of cultural differences on the identification of learning disabilities.

☞   Discuss the skills involved in the integration of speech/special education services with mainstream curriculum and instruction.

☞   Develop an understanding of the significant advantages of a whole-language approach in working with children with language disorders in an inclusive classroom setting.

Critical Concepts

Section:

Definitions

Concept:

Several types of learning disabilities may be observed in school aged children and youth. Each has clinically observable and distinguishing characteristics. Congress enacted public law (94-142 and 99-457) to define and to enhance public education for disabled students, including children with specific learning disabilities. The federal definition was challenged by professionals from the private sector who advocated emphasis on the heterogeneity of learning disabilities.

1.   How may learning disabilities manifested in the classroom?

2.   List the other names given in the text by which learning disabilities have been known:

3.   What conditions are ruled out of the category of learning disabilities?

4.   Contrast the federal definition of learning disability with that of the NJCLD.

5.   What is the range of estimated prevalence of learning disabled students in school aged children?

6.   Describe the clinical characteristics of the following learning disability syndromes.

      A.   Language disorder syndrome:

      B.   Graphomotor discoordination syndrome:

      C.   Visuospatial perceptual deficit syndrome:

      D.   Attention deficit disorder (with or without hyperactivity):

      E.   Nonverbal learning disabilities:

7.   List four factors that influence the outcome of learning disabilities.

      A.

      B.

      C.

D.

8.   What is a *genetic* cause of disability? List the two confirmed genetic causes of learning disability.

A.

B.

Section:

Underlying mechanisms

Concept:

Advances in the knowledge of the relationship between brain physiology and behavior has implicated several neurological sites as sources of learning disability. Research has associated abnormal structure of dominant hemisphere language centers, subcortical structures and familial patterns in dysfunctional language development. Language learning abnormalities may also be caused by exogenous factors, such as brain injury.

1.   What parts of the brain have been associated with activating attention?

A.

B.

2.   What is the evidence of cerebral cortical involvement in learning disabilities?

Section:

Examples and Characteristics

Concept:

To learn the complexities of adult language children must employ their highest intellectual functions. For most, this process is a natural human growth process. For children with a learning disability, successful language use presents a special challenge that affects their personality adjustment, school performance and life activities. Children must develop metalinguistic skills that allow them to conceive and manipulate language. They must also develop language strategies based on communication scenarios they encounter as they grow.

1.   What are the three steps in the "communication game?"

   A.

   B.

   C.

2.   List five characteristics of communication expertise:

   A.

   B.

   C.

   D.

E.

3.   List the developmental prerequisites for communication strategy use that are acquired at the following ages:

    A.   Ages five to seven:

        I.

        ii.

    B.   Ages seven to thirteen:

    C.   Ages eight to fifteen:

3.   What strategic communication difficulties would you expect of a language-learning disabled child of age fifteen?

4.   What three types of *scripts* did Schrank (1990) identify?

    A.

    B.

C.

5.   How may a language learning disability affect a student's pragmatic communication skills?

6.   What are nonverbal communication patterns that may affect the pragmatic communication strategies of the language-learning disabled student?

7.   Name six word learning differences or difficulties encountered by language-learning disabled students.

A.

B.

C.

D.

E.

F.

8.   Pick a word (*Write it here:* _____) and describe its eight semantic cues as listed in the text:

A.   Class Membership:

131

B.   Causal Attributes:

C.   Spatial Attributes:

D.   Temporal Attributes:

E.   Value:

F.   Stative Descriptive Attributes:

G.   Functional Descriptive Attributes:

H.   Equivalence:

9.   List two reasons for the language learning disabled child to use prototypical, simple forms for communication. What difficulties might this cause?

A.

B.

10.   List seven characteristics of brain injury in children (after Ylvisaker and Gobble, 1987).

A.

B.

C.

D.

E.

F.

G.

11.   What additional problem do children with language-learning disabilities have when English is not their primary language?

Section:

Assessment Approaches and Strategies

Concept:

Evaluating language and communication is like a detective game. The student's case must be examined from several viewpoints, with several methods, and at several opportunities. The detective game continues with observations fot eh child while treatment is ongoing.

1.   Describe the advantages of a norm-referenced instrument.

2.   List the four purposes of norm-referenced assessment.

A.

B.

133

C.

D.

2. What is the difference between a criterion-referenced assessment instrument and a norm-referenced instrument?

3. List the four purposes of a criterion-referenced assessment.

    A.

    B.

    C.

    D.

4. List the three purposes of observational ratings and interviews.

    A.

    B.

C.

5. What is a prortfolio-based assessment?

6. List the dimensions of Wiig's and Story's (1993) S-MAP portfolio assessment.

A.

B.

C.

D.

E.

7. After traumatic brain injury, what four areas should be examined?

A.

B.

C.

D.

Section:

Intervention Perspectives

Concept:

Language perspective has shifted from emphasis on grammatical rules and forms to focus on context and function. Accordingly, intervention in language disabilities has shifted emphasis from isolation of the indidividual and the disability to inclusion of the student in the regular clasrooms. Speech-language pathologists collaborate and consult with teachers to create a classroom language environment that utilizes and stimulates the student's strengths.

1.   How does *inclusion* lessen the restrictions on a language-challenged student's learning environment?

2.   List three principles of a whole language approach.

         A.

         B.

         C.

3.   What is the diference between *collaboration* and *consultation*?

4.   List the professions that should be involved in the treatment of a child with a language - learning disability.

5.   Describe the trajectory of strategy-based intervention.

6.   How can strategy-based language intervention help a language-learning disabled child in daily life?

7.   List three benefits of counseling for the child with language-learning disability.

      A.

      B.

      C.

Critical Terms

Define the following terms, using your text as a reference:

o Aphasia

o Attention Deficit Disorder

o Articulatory and Graphomotor Dyscoordination Syndrome

o Attention Deficit-Hyperactivity Disorder

o Learning Disability

o Language Learning Disability

o Fragile X Syndrome

o Turner Syndrome

o Strategic Functioning

o Cortical

o Subcortical

o Norm-Referenced Assessment

o Criterion-Referenced Assessment

o Portfolio Assessment

o Script Knowledge

o Code-Switching

o Nonverbal Learning

o Whole-Language

o Scaffolding

o   Scripts

o   Whole-Language Approach

o   Social Drama

o   Public Law 94-142

o   Inclusion

Chapter Six Self Test

True/False

1. A child cannot learn to read or write fluently if the native language has not been learned adequately.
    > True
    > False

2. By legal definition, children with learning disabilities have problems in all academic areas.
    > True
    > False

3. There is a high incidence of brain injury among children with LLD.
    > True
    > False

4. The most common learning disability syndrome is termed *language disorder syndrome* (language-learning disabilities).
    > True
    > False

5. If intervention has not begun by third grade, it is to late to help the LLD child.
    > True
    > False

6. Language learning disabilities may appear in 5% of all children diagnosed as learning disabled.
    > True
    > False

7. Children and adolescents with *visuospatial perceptual deficit syndrome* have difficulty with visually oriented tasks.
    > True
    > False

8. Children with ADD may not be hyperactive.
    > True
    > False

9. Nondominant hemisphere dysfunction may affect reasoning, social perception and inner language
    > True
    > False

10. Learning disabilities have no genetic basis.
    > True
    > False

11. The primary language processing area in the left cerebral hemisphere is known as Wernicke's area.
    True
    False

12. Once a child grows into adolescence, it is too late for effective language therapy.
    True
    False

13. Children with language-learning disabilities often have difficulty recognizing verbal patterns in communication.
    True
    False

14. Classroom scripts develop in an ongoing process.
    True
    False

15. Children with language disabilities generally have difficulty with text comprehension.
    True
    False

16. Children with LLD may earn lower grades because they lack the ability to control narrative structure.
    True
    False

17. It would not be unusual for a student with LLD to score normally on a picture vocabulary test.
    True
    False

18. Traumatic brain injury may disrupt use of all acquired linguistic skills.
    True
    False

19. Most immigrants and persons from culturally diverse backgrounds display characteristics of language-learning disabilities.
    True
    False

20. Portfolio assessment is a form of performance assessment.
    True
    False

21. Strategy-based intervention uses passive techniques.
    True
    False

22. Students with LLD use common scripts for daily life functions, but must be supported to recognize classroom scripts.
    True
    False

23. Whole-language approaches emphasize choosing one language modality appropriate to a communicative situation.
    True
    False

24. Language intervention should be the only treatment required for language learning deficits.
    True
    False

25. The inclusion movement emphasizes that teachers must help students develop self-image.
    True
    False

Multiple Choice

1. Language learning disabilities may affect performance in which of the following areas?
    a. listening
    b. speaking
    c. writing
    d. all of the above

2. The least common deficit syndrome among children and adolescents with specific learning disability is:
    a. visuospatial perceptual deficit
    b. articulatory and graphomotor dyscoordination syndrome
    c. sensory-motor deficit
    d. language learning disabilities

3. Which area of the brain is primarily implicated in attention deficit disorder?
    a. frontal lobe
    b. parietal lobe
    c. occipital lobe
    d. temporal lobe

4. Which of the following genetic disorders is associated with learning disabilities?
    a. Turner syndrome
    b. Marfan's syndrome
    c. Hunter's syndrome
    d. Down syndrome

5. Electrical stimulation of which part of the brain produced disruptions in speech sound discrimination in Ojemann and Mateer's (1979) study?
    a. corpus striatum
    b. left temporal lobe
    c. right temporal lobe
    d. thalamus
6. Nonverbal learning disabilities are characterized by:
    a. deficient math and reasoning skills
    b. poor visuospatial, organizational, and social perception skills
    c. inadequate social skills
    d. all of the above
7. When LLD is precipitated by a traumatic brain injury, the disability is said to be:
    a. syndromic
    b. biological
    c. transient
    d. acquired
8. Which of the following skills is required to use language as a joke?
    a. metalinguistic
    b. paralinguistic
    c. visual closure
    d. figure-ground discrimination
9. At what age should a child appropriately interpret figurative word use?
    a. two years
    b. five years
    c. thirteen years
    d. eighteen years
10. Which of the following is among the prerequisites for communication strategy use?
    a. ability to substitute words
    b. ability to switch codes
    c. ability to inhibit responses and reflect
    d. ability to circumlocute
11. Children with language-learning disabilities often progress to the linguistic transition stages typical for which ages?
    a. three to five years
    b. seven to ten years
    c. ten to fifteen years
    d. fifteen to twenty years
12. The underlying plan of a conversation is called a...
    a. speech
    b. script
    c. poem
    d. billet doux

13. Stubbs (1993) found which of the following among the cohesive mechanisms for discourse and narrative?
     a. use of synonyms
     b. verbal math skills
     c. ability to follow lexical repetition patterns
     d. ability to associate a word with a picture

14. Which of the following is the best single indicator of reading achievement?
     a. word knowledge
     b. sequential memory
     c. pragmatic skills
     d. nonverbal communication

15. What type of word task might we expect to present difficulty to a child with LLD?
     a. matching spoken words to pictures
     b. remembering series of spoken words
     c. saying the antonyms of spoken words
     d. rhyming spoken words

16. Which of the following semantic cues is/are required for a student to learn the meaning of a new word from text?
     a. its class membership
     b. its spelling
     c. articulatory posture of its initial sound
     d. all of the above

17. In addition to language therapy, the child with LLD is most likely to need what other type of treatment?
     a. physical therapy
     b. occupational therapy
     c. nursing
     d. counseling

18. A mature language user responds to perceived needs of listeners through which process?
     a. direction
     b. metalinguistic ability
     c. paraphrasing
     d. manners

19. The most common effects of closed head injury result from damage to which nervous system structure?
     a. Wernicke's area
     b. Broca's area
     c. basal ganglia
     d. A single focal site usually cannot be identified

20. Which of the following is a useful communication strategy for students with LLD?
    a. use pictures for redundancy
    b. speak very slowly
    c. use multiple words with the same meaning
    d. reduce complex pragmatic rules to simple, automated ones

21. The counseling approach in which the counselor shares knowledge to increase the client's understanding is called what?
    a. direct approach
    b. indirect approach
    c. self-oriented approach
    d. treatment oriented approach

22. Wernicke's area is located in the:
    a. subcortical region
    b. cerebral cortex
    c. spinal cord
    d. lateral geniculate nucleus

23. Which of the following is an outcome of norm-referenced testing?
    a. Determination of language disability presence
    b. Identify strengths and weaknesses
    c. Determine eligibility for placement
    d. all of the above

24. Criterion referenced testing can be used to...
    a. determine placement eligibility
    b. compare the subject's performance to a large sample of other children
    c. verify results of norm-referenced testing
    d. determine the presence of a language disability

Chapter Seven Students' Guide

Phonological Disorders

Richard G. Schwartz

Chapter Summary

The purpose of this chapter is to examine approaches to understanding the nature, assessment, and remediation of phonological disorders. By providing a detailed overview of the theoretical bases of phonological acquisition and disorders, and the nature of disorders the chapter presents a solid framework for the understanding of phonological development and it's implications for the Speech-Language Pathologist.

Student Outcomes

After reading this chapter students should be able to:

☞ Discuss information on the nature and causes of phonological disorders.

☞ Compare and contrast a variety of approaches in the assessment of phonological disorders.

☞ Compare and contrast a variety of approaches to the treatment of phonological disorders.

☞ Discuss specific procedures for summarizing phonological error patterns in oral language.

☞ Distinguish between *phonological* and *phonetic* disorders.

Critical Concepts

Section:

Introduction

Concept:

Phonology is the study of that aspect of language that includes consonants, vowels and syllables and the linguistic rules that govern their combinations. In speech-language pathology, the term phonology *has subsumed the domain of* articulation. *Phonological disorders are the most common of children who have a communication disorder.*

1.   What is unique about phonology among the other aspects of language?

2.   How does phonology differ from writing?

Section:

The nature of phonological disorders

Concept:

Phonological disorders are distinct from phonetic disorders. While both include perceptual and production components, the essence of a phonological disorder lies in the cognitive-linguistic aspect of spoken language.

1.   What professional confirms the presence of a phonological disorder?

2.   What two considerations are important in the clinical approach to a phonological disorder?

   A.

   B.

3. Describe a *mild* phonological disorder.

4. Describe a severe phonological disorder.

5. What are the three levels of the phonological system?

    A.

    B.

    C.

6. For the following conditions, indicate whether they are phonological or phonetic:

    A. Apraxia

    B. Consistent productions of /w/ in the place of /r/

    C. Deletion of final unstressed syllables

    D. Nasalization of all speech sounds due to velopharyngeal paralysis

7. List four characteristics of high level phonological disorders.

    A.

    B.

    C.

    D.

8. Describe two differences between normally developing children with immature phonology and children who have phonological disorders.

    A.

B.

Section:

Determinants of Phonological Disorders

Concept:

Phonological disorders may result from many cognitive or physical etiological factors, singly or in combination.

1.   Give two clinically important reasons to investigate the determinants of phonological disorders?

A.

B.

Section:

Motor Abilities

Concept:

Oral motor abilities appear to be related to speech motor movements in a complex fashion. Children may have speech motor difficulties in the absence of general motor problems, and non-speech movements of the oral mechanism are different in origin and function than speech movements.

1.   How is diadochokinesis typically assessed?

2.   Why should/should not speech-language pathologists include tongue thrust treatment to correct /s/ and /z/ distortions?

3.   What characteristic would distinguish a child with developmental apraxia from children who have phonological disorders?

Section:

Speech Perception and Audition

Concept:

Although the relationship between speech perception and production is not fully understood, it seems clear that normal hearing is important to the acquisition of normal phonology. Individual children will demonstrate unique phonological characteristics based upon their personal abilities, developmental stage and auditory functions.

1.   What are two important factors determining the extent of phonological deficits in children with hearing impairments?

       A.

       B.

2.   Which speech sounds are least visible?

3.   Which aspects of speech are least salient perceptually?

4.   How did Otitis Media affect phonology in the children studied by the author of the chapter?

Section:

Dentition

Concept:

Dentition may be implicated in a minority of speech articulation problems.

1.   Should a child with missing upper incisors who misarticulates /s/ be considered for speech therapy? Why?

Section:

Intelligence

Concept:

General developmental delays, such as those manifested in Down syndrome, appear to affect phonological development as they affect other functions.

1.   Describe the author's observations on the phonology of children with Down Syndrome.

Section:

Language

Concept:

Phonological developmental delays sometimes accompany delays in general linguistic development. This relationship may be attributed to the close tie between phonology speech grammatical morphology and because of the effects of increasing linguistic complexity that accompanies maturation. Children who have difficulty with grammatical morphemes may need direct phonological intervention to accompany their focus on syntax.

1. What phonological segments denote *plurality* in English?

2. Describe the relationship between phonological complexity and syntactic complexity.

3. What is the relationship between speech articulation and the acquisition of *new information?*

Section:

Reading

Concept:

The relationship between written letters and spoken sounds places increasing demands on the child's ability to consider phonology as an entity in itself. Children who have difficulty with manipulating phonology or who have short term memory delays are likely to have difficulty reading.

1. What is the relationship between metalinguistic ability and metaphonological ability?

2. Why should short term memory be important to phonology and to reading?

Section:

Assessment

Concept:

Three phases of assessment carry the process of intervention in phonological disorders from identification to ongoing discharge. Several components of assessment include observations of the child's phonological behavior in several contexts, study of the case history, and examination of orofacial anatomy and physiology.

1. What are the goal of the following phases of assessment?

   A. Screening:

   B. Identification:

   C. Diagnosis:

2. When a child "fails" a screening, what is the implication?

3. List six important items in the case history of a child with a suspected phonological disorder.

   A.

B.

C.

D.

E.

F.

Section:

Sampling and Analyzing Children's Speech

Concept:

Several formats for sampling a child's speech involve a variety of contexts. Each has its advantages in developing a diagnostic impression about the structure of the child's phonology.

1.   Write the unique advantages of the following published articulation tests.

A.   *Goldman-Fristoe Test of Articulation:*

B.   *Fisher-Logemann Test of Articulation Competence:*

C.   *Photo Articulation Test:*

D.   *Templin-Darley Tests of Articulation:*

E.   *Arizona Articulation Proficiency Scale:*

155

F. *Kahn-Lewis Phonological Analysis:*

G. *The Assessment of Phonological Processes-Revised (Hodson):*

2. What are the advantages of an articulation test?

3. What are three general limitations of published articulation tests?

   A.

   B.

   C.

4. What should a clinician bear in mind about the target words of a speech articulation test?

5. Name three ways to facilitate the speech sampling procedure.

   A.

B.

C.

6. What is the major disadvantage of the speech sample?

7. What is the advantage of an elicited speech sample?

8. Why is phonetic transcription necessary when we have electronic recording devices?

9. Distinguish between an independent sample analysis and a relational sample analysis?

10. What should the clinician look for in an independent analysis?

11.   What is the overall goal of the sample analysis?

Section:

Perception testing

Concept:

Some children with phonological disorders may have auditory perceptual disorders as well. The clinician is advised to study the case history and use special tests to determine the role of auditory perception in a case of disordered phonology.

1.   How can a clinician design a test suited to a particular child's phonology?

Section:

Oral Mechanism Examination; Audiological Testing

Concept:

Clinicians should examine the form and function of the speech mechanism to develop a full concept of the basis for a phonological disorder. An audiologist should evaluate the hearing of children with speech disorders.

1.   Describe the physical structures examined in the oral mechanism.

2.   Describe the functions that speech-language pathologists should examine in the evaluation of the oral mechanism.

3.   Why should a phonologically disordered child have an audiological evaluation?

Sections:

Stimulability; Determining Intelligibility

Concept:

Clinicians facilitate the remediation process by assessing stimulability for therapeutic stimuli and my measuring speech intelligibility.

1.   How does a clinician determine if a child is *stimulable*?

2.   What is the purpose of intelligibility rating?

Section:

The Process of Assessment

Concept:

There is an orderly flow to the process of assessment.

1.   Describe the process of assessment following referral by screening.

2.   Why have clinicians begun to avoid age-referenced norms?

3.   What are the author's suggested norm-referenced criteria for determining the presence of a disorder?

      A.   Percentile?

      B.   Z-Scores (Standard Deviations)?

4.   How can a speech-language pathologist avoid dialect reduction as a goal in phonological treatment?

Section:

Intervention

Concept:

The speech-language pathologist approaches intervention with a framework appropriate to the particular case at hand. The intervention process in phonological disorders begins with a statement of the child's initial level of phonological function and details of therapeutic goals and objectives. The plan of treatment begins by training the child to perform the targeted phonological function and ends when the child demonstrates assimilation of that function.

1.   Why does a clinician create a facilitating context at the beginning of treatment?

Section:

Articulation Approaches

Concept:

Articulation focus on motor production, using operant principles to reinforce establishment of the target behavior as a phonological entity. The articulation approaches may be best suited for children whose errors do not seem to reflect underlying deficits in phonology.

1.   What distinguishes the "Articulation" approach to treatment?

2.   Describe these steps in the "Traditional" articulation approach:

    A.   "Ear training"

B.   "Production training"

3.   What are the steps in the "Multiple Phonemic" approach of McCabe and Bradley (1975) ?

A.

B.

C.

4.   Winitz (1969) stressed the role of speech discrimination training. Does such an approach belong in the "Articulation" category or in the "Phonological" category of intervention?

Section:

Phonological Approaches

Concept:

Speech-language pathologists have been slow to develop treatment paradigms consistent with the cognitive-linguistic framework of phonological function they have so readily accepted.

1.   What was the premise of the Distinctive Feature approaches developed in the 1970's?

2.   List the five assumptions implicit in the "Cycles" approach of Hodson and Paden (1991).

   A.

   B.

   C.

   D.

   E.

3. How is the "Minimal Pair" or "Contrast" approach similar to Winitz' (1969) approach?

4. Why might a "phonological" approach be most suitable for a child with unintelligible conversational speech.

Section:

Frequency and General Organization of Therapy

Concept:

Treatment frequency and environment should be targeted for the individual child and that child's stage in therapy.

1. What are three determinants of treatment schedules for phonological therapy?

   A.

   B.

   C.

2. Describe three ways in which multiple phonological goals are addressed in therapy. According to the author, which way most closely resembles normal acquisition?

   A.

   B.

C.

Sections:

Measuring Change; Criteria; Determining the Source of Change

Concept:

One of the most important skills of the clinical speech-language pathologist is the establishment of criteria for progression to more complex treatment activities or for dismissal from treatment altogether. Changes must be measured with attention to stimulus context and response type. Clinicians are interested in determining the source of phonological change so they may modify their approaches to a given child's treatment as indicated.

1.   Which criteria would you choose: 90% or 60% mastery in conversation?

2.   What does self-correction in speech suggest?

3.   How do clinicians support the contention that phonological change is probably an effect of treatment and not spontaneous?

Sections:

Intervention Settings; Generalization

Concept:

The best setting for treatment depends upon the particular child and may change as treatment progresses.

1. What are the advantages and disadvantages of individual treatment versus group treatment?

2. Describe what Fey (1986) might consider the most and least natural aspects of the following aspects of therapy.

    A. Treatment Activities:

        i.   Most natural

        ii. Least Natural

    B. Physical Context:

        i.   Most natural

        ii. Least Natural

    C. Social Context:

        i.   Most natural

        ii. Least Natural

Critical Terms

Define the following terms, using your text as a reference:

o   Articulation

o   Organic Disorder

o   Phonological Disorder

o   Chronic Otitis Media

o   Baseline

o   Independent Sample Analyses

o   Establishment

o   Successive Approximations

o   Auditory Bombardment

o   Control Goals

o   Phonology

o   Functional Disorders

o   Diadichokinesis

o   Malocclusion

o   Phonetic Inventory

o   Relational Sample Analyses

o   Generalization

o   Distinctive Features

o   Multiple Baseline Data

- o   Intelligibility

- o   Phonetic Disorder

- o   Tongue Thrust

- o   Minimal Pairs

- o   Phonological Processes

- o   Stimulability

- o   Maintenance

- o   Cycle Approach

- o   Target Goals

Chapter Five Self Test

True/False

1. Articulation is not a part of phonology.
   - True
   - False
2. For the best assessment of a child's phonological skills, a speech-language pathologist should look at syllable formation in a variety of contexts
   - True
   - False
3. A disorder of the motor production system is likely to produce a phonetic disorder
   - True
   - False
4. For many children, phonological disorders are accompanied by syntactic deficits.
   - True
   - False
5. Intelligibility refers to how well a child's speech is understood.
   - True
   - False
6. Phonological disabilities in children with hearing disorders varies with the type and severity of the loss.
   - True
   - False
7. There is no relationship between intelligence and intelligibility.
   - True
   - False
8. A phonological disorder is a sure sign of other developmental disorders.
   - True
   - False
9. Research suggests that children produce nouns more accurately than they produce verbs.
   - True
   - False
10. Reading seems to be dependent on metaphonological abilities.
    - True
    - False
11. Signs of general sensory deficits are of no significance in assessment of phonology.
    - True
    - False

12. Commercially available articulation tests are advantageous in cases where the child's speech is very unintelligible.

     True

     False

13. Phonology describes the contrastive elements in written language.

     True

     False

14. Some children have different sound-contrast systems than adults.

     True

     False

15. Phonological development stabilized at age five.

     True

     False

16. A child who "fails" a screening is referred for evaluation.

     True

     False

17. Most standardized tests allow for cultural variations in children's responses.

     True

     False

18. Phonological disorders are sure signs of perceptual disorders.

     True

     False

19. Any child being evaluated for a phonological disorder should receive a complete audiological evaluation.

     True

     False

20. The maintenance phase of articulation treatment addresses production in conversational speech.

     True

     False

21. Early forms of phonological treatment focused on distinctive feature training.

     True

     False

22. The "cycle" approach sets no performance criteria before progression to the next goal.

     True

     False

23. Therapy frequency may be dictated by the clinician's schedule.

     True

     False

24. The speech-language pathologist may be considered a natural interactor under most circumstances.

     True

     False

25. Effective treatment activities must provide the child opportunities to hear correct responses.

      True

      False

Multiple Choice.

1. Which of the following describes *phonology*?
      a the structure of conversation
      b. the meaning of words and larger units
      c. the structure of words in terms of consonants, vowels, and syllables
      d. the structure of complex words and inflections

2. Children who have phonological disorders have:
      a. hearing impairments
      b. structural anomalies
      c. motor disorders
      d. linguistic deficits

3. Phonological disorders are characterized by :
      a. widespread patterns of errors
      b. limitations on syllable structure
      c. limitations in the range of sounds produced
      d. all of the above

4. Rapid utterance of a series of syllables is called...
      a. diadochokinesis
      b. imitative movement
      c. blathering
      d. balanced movement

5. Clinicians approach "tongue thrust" as a...
      a. phonological disorder
      b. phonetic disorder
      c. swallowing disorder
      d. syntactical disorder

6. What is the assumed underlying disability in *developmental apraxia of speech*?
      a. paralysis
      b. linguistic disturbance
      c. auditory perceptual disorder
      d. sequencing motor movements

7. What is the relationship between otitis media and phonological disorders?
      a. it is the number one cause of phonological disorder
      b. it has no effect on speech development
      c. the relationship is not clear
      d. none of the above

8.   In phonological assessment when does diagnosis occur?
     a.   during the screening process
     b.   after identification
     c.   after a period of treatment
     d.   six months after screening

9.   Which of the following is an advantage of commercially available articulation tests?
     a.   They provide analysis of phonological systems.
     b.   They provide a natural context for evaluation
     c.   They provide a way to compare unintelligible speech to the adult target.
     d.   They have no advantages.

10. The *Kahn-Lewis Phonological Analysis* is intended to be used with which commercial articulation test?
     a.   all articulation tests
     b.   *Fisher-Logemann Test of Articulation Competence*
     c.   *Arizona Articulation Proficiency Scale*
     d.   *Goldman-Fristoe Test of Articulation*

11. Independent phonological analysis examines a child's...
     a.   phonetic inventory
     b.   phonological processes
     c.   approximations of the adult target
     d.   distinctive feature analysis

12. Which of the following is inferred through phonological sample analysis?
     a.   the child's knowledge of phonology
     b.   the child's perceptual abilities
     c.   the child's phonetic production abilities
     d.   all of the above

13. What is the anterior one-third of the palate called?
     a.   hard palate
     b.   soft palate
     c.   buccal cavity
     d.   fistulae

14. What does stimulability for syllables in an imitative context reflect?
     a.   phonetic level perception
     b.   phonological knowledge
     c.   phonological representation
     d.   phonological organization

15. What purpose may be served by intelligibility assessment?
     a.   establishment of a measure of functional effects
     b.   provides a diversion for the child
     c.   may predict the outcome of treatment
     d.   aids in intelligence assessment

16. Which of the following is the goal of *generalization* in therapy?
    a. ensure motoric competence
    b. ensure perceptual ability
    c. establishment of the phonological act
    d. ensure changes are systemic phonologically

17. A relational sample analysis is an examination of...
    a. the relationships between a child's productions in different contexts.
    b. the relationship between the child's production and characteristics of the adult target.
    c. the relationship between the adult target and the treatment objective.
    d. the relationship between the child and the clinician.

18. What are the focuses of "articulation" approaches to treatment?
    a. cognitive structure
    b. phonological abilities
    c. motor production
    d. phonological acquisition

19. When should a child be dismissed from therapy?
    a. when speech is 100% intelligible.
    b. when all goals have been reached at the established criterion level
    c. after six months
    d. when the child reaches age twelve

20. Which of the following is one of Fey's (1986) dimensions of naturalness?
    a. treatment materials
    b. vocal characteristics
    c. physical context
    d. standardization sample

Chapter Eight Students' Guide

Voice Disorders

Douglas M. Hicks

Chapter Summary

People are identified and associated with their individual voice characteristics, yet most people do not consider voice disorders to be a serious speech problem. The voice is the most often used sound source for speech, important in the formation of all vowels, semivowels and voiced obstruent consonants. Phonation, or the production of the voice, is a function of the larynx, gateway to the respiratory system. Specialists in voice disorders are familiar with the anatomical and physiological dimensions of voice production and disorders. Voice disorders may result from faulty phonatory habits or from disease. Treatment of cancer of the larynx may require removal of the larynx to save the life of the patient. The speech-language pathologist must then teach the patient how to use alternate phonatory sources. The assessment and clinical management of voice disorders is an important aspect of speech-language pathology

Student Outcomes

After reading this chapter students should be able to do the following:

☞ Differentiate between the characteristics of a NORMAL and DISORDERED voice.

☞ Relate perceptual and physical characteristics of the glottal tone, including: Pitch/Frequency; Loudness/Amplitude; and Quality/Complexity (Spectrum).

☞ Discuss ORGANIC and NONORGANIC factors related to voice disorders.

☞ Discuss methodologies involved in the assessment of the voice.

☞ Discuss treatment considerations for the voice client.

175

Section:

Voice Problems Among Communication Disorders

Concept:

Deviations of pitch, loudness or quality in a person's voice is evidence of a voice disorder. It is difficult to state definitively what constitutes a disordered voice and just as difficult to estimate the prevalence of voice disorders. Those seeking the services of a speech-language pathologist for help with voice problems usually do so when they perceive a threat to their social acceptance or income.

1. How does a speech-language pathologist distinguish an "abnormal" voice from a "normal" one?

2. Why do people rarely pay attention to phonatory disorders?

3. What are some occupations that require a normal sounding voice?

Section:

Phonation and the Larynx

Concept:

Normal phonation depends on smooth, regular functioning of the vocal folds.

1.   Describe what is meant by "smooth"\function of the vocal folds.

Section:

Parallel Perceptual and Physical Factors

Concept:

The normal voice is a quasi periodic, complex sound. The physical measurements associated with any sound may be associated with certain psychological characteristics that are not so easily measured.

1.   What *pitch*?

2.   How is pitch changed by a singer?

3.   What is volume-velocity?

4.   How is greater subglottal air pressure associated with loudness in the voice?

5.   Is the normal voice comprised of more than one tone?

6.   What is the role of noise in normal speech?

Section:

Resonance

Concept:

Coupling of the larynx with the cavities of the throat and head, alters the quality of the laryngeal tone through acoustic resonance. A speaker may change the resonating characteristics of the vocal tract by contracting the muscles of the pharynx and oral cavity. This action is the basis for vowel formation. Disease may affect the resonating characteristics of the vocal tract by changing the vibratory actions of the vocal folds or by changing in the flexibility of the vocal tract walls.

1.   What does the author mean by enhancement or repression if *partials*?

2.   What is the effect of an open velopharyngeal port?

3.   What effect does an extra mass, such as a polyp, have on vocal fold vibration? What effect does it have on vocal tract resonance?

4.   What wold be the effect of introducing another vibrator or sound generator into a normal vocal tract?

Section:

Factors that Influence Vocal Fold Vibration and Voice

Concept:

The voice may be affected by nonorganic factors and by organic factors. These factors affect the voice by altering vocal fold adduction, mass, tension or subglottic air pressure. Nonorganic causes arise from psychological factors. Organic conditions arise from paralysis, growth of excess tissue or injury.

1.   What is the difference between *aphonia* and *dysphonia*?

2.   What events might cause aphonia?

3.   What is the relationship between the speech-language pathologist and the physician in the treatment of organic voice disorders?

4.   Why might bilateral vocal fold paralysis be a threat to a patient's life?

5.   What other organic factors might impair vocal fold adduction?

6.   Describe the effects of trauma to the laryngeal cartilages on vocal fold vibration.

7.   How can blood deficiency affect phonation?

8.   Why does the presence of a protruding mass affect the quality of the voice?

Section:

Localized Lesions and Other Disorders

Concept:

There are several conditions in which abnormal tissue growth, called neoplasm, compromises the function of the larynx. Benign neoplasms are bothersome, but affect only laryngeal function. The prognosis for recovery is favorable. Malignant neoplasms can be life threatening. Recovery from these may depend on medical treatment.

1.   List Aronson's (1990) effects of mass lesions on vocal function.

      A.

      B.

      C.

D.

E.

F.

2.   Describe the role of the speech-language pathologist in diagnosing mass lesions of the vocal folds.

3.   List five benign neoplasms of the larynx.

A.

B.

C.

D.

E.

4.   What is the usual cause of vocal fold nodules?

5.   Who has the responsibility for treatment of laryngeal carcinoma?

Section:

Voice Disorders Related to Resonance Deviations

Concept:

Too much or too little nasal resonance is the source of most voice resonance disorders. Treatment of voice disorders involves the distinction of the role of resonance disorders from that of phonatory disorders.

1.   What organic conditions cause hypernasality?

      A.

      B.

2.   How can *dialect* contribute to the perception of hypernasality?

3.   What are "adenoids," and what is their role in resonance? *(Hint: consult an anatomy text to answer this question.)*

Section:

Assessment and Diagnosis

Concept:

There is no "best" system of voice assessment and diagnosis, but the author's five-step plan is a good structure for clinical practice.

1. List the five steps of the author's assessment and diagnosis plan. Of what value is each step in the treatment of voice disorders?

    A.

    B.

    C.

    D.

    E.

2. What is the voice pathologist's most useful skill?

3. Of what use is the sound recorder in the "listening" phase of voice evaluation?

4. By the time the voice pathologist has listened to voice samples, what should she/he be able to describe?

5. What is the purpose of "looking" in assessment of a voice disorder?

6. List the five types of information to be obtained by examining the case history.

    A.

    B.

    C.

    D.

7. What family factors should the voice pathologist consider in the evaluation of voice disorders?

8. List three points that the clinician should include in the voice evaluation report.

    A.

    B.

    C.

Section:

Therapy for Voice Disorders

Concept:

Therapy for voice disorders intervenes in the overall health of the patient with a combination of medical, environmental and direct approaches. The extent to which each approach plays a role in treatment depends upon the peculiarities of each case.

1.   What therapies comprise the medical approach to voice therapy?

      A.

      B.

      C.

2.   How can environmental manipulation help a voice problem?

3.   List the seven components of the direct approach to voice therapy.

      A.

      B.

      C.

      D.

      E.

      F.

      G.

      H.

4. What is the first important step in listening for voice therapy?

5. Describe what the author means when he writes of "mental hygiene."

6. Under what circumstances should a speech-language pathologist undertake the role of psychological counselor?

7. What are the author's presumptions underlying his emphasis on physical well-being?

8. How can poor posture and limited movement influence voice production?

9. Why is breathing important to good voice production?

10. Describe the four approaches to relaxation.

    A.

    B.

    C.

D.

11.   What are the six components of direct voice training?

A.

B.

C.

D.

E.

F.

12.   Can eliminating vocal abuse also be included in the "environmental" or "mental hygiene" approaches?

13.   At what point does the average voice reach its optimum pitch?

14.   What is the purpose of the drill during which the patient repeats, "How high is the house? How does that drill achieve such a purpose?

15.   What are some reasons for modifying a person's habitual vocal pitch?

16.   What are four reasons a person may speak with insufficient loudness?

    A.

    B.

    C.

    D.

17.   How does one increase the Bernoulli effect in the laryngopharynx?

18.   If exercises fail, what is another option for increasing vocal loudness?

19.   What is the author's analogy between tennis and voice building?

20.   How is vocal resonance modified?

21. What are the most obvious resonance disorders?

Section:

Speech Without a Larynx

Concept:

Some patients with cancer or severe injury must undergo a laryngectomy as a means of survival. This surgical procedure removes the natural phonatory source from the vocal tract, and speech therapy involves teaching the patient how to use an alternate source.

1. What are three alternate phonatory sources available to laryngectomees?

   A.

   B.

   C.

2. What separates are the airway and the food-fluid channels in the laryngectomy procedure? Why?

3. What are the power sources of available artificial larynges?

4.   How do the two variations of electronic transfer acoustic energy to the oral cavity?

5.   What two anatomical passages are bridged by surgically implanted artificial larynges? How do they transfer acoustic energy into the vocal tract?

6.   What is the longest duration a surgically implanted artificial larynx remain in place?

7.   What is the most frustrating problem for alaryngeal speakers?

Critical Terms

Define the following terms, using your text as a reference:

o   Aphonia

o   Dysphonia

o   Voice Disorder

o   Glissando

o   Nasal Twang

o   Hypernasality

o   Hyponasality

o   Pitch

o   Frequency

o   Amplitude

o   Complexity

o   Resonance

o   Hyperfunctional Dysphonia

o   Contact Ulcer

o   Ankylosis

o   Anemia

o   Myasthenia

o   Polyp

o   Vocal Nodules

- o Papillomata

- o Carcinoma

- o Edema

- o Laryngeal Web

- o Cyst

- o Laryngectomy

- o Esophageal Speech

- o Alaryngeal Speech

- o Stoma

- o P-E Segment

- o Progressive Relaxation

- o Differential Relaxation

- o Optimum Pitch

Chapter Eight Self Test

True/False

1. The vocal folds are adducted during quiet respiration.
    True
    False

2. Stutterng is a voice disorder.
    True
    False

3. Vowel contrasts are created by resonance variations.
    True
    False

4. Without a functinal larynx, speech is impossible.
    True
    False

5. All males have roughly the same optimum vocal pitch..
    True
    False

6. Changes in vocal fold mass can affect the sond of the voice.
    True
    False

7. A change in amplitude produces a change in pitch.
    True
    False

8. Most phonemes require a phonatory source.
    True
    False

9. Aphonia is the complete loss of voice.
    True
    False

10. Bilateral vocal fold paralysis is a threat to the patient's airway.
    True
    False

11. In the total laryngectomy procedure, the surgeon creates a new airway.
    True
    False

12. Each neoplasm of thelarynx creates a distinct sound, enabling accurate acoustic diagnosis.
    True
    False

13. The vocal folds produce a complex sound.
    True
    False

14. Subglottic air pressure is related to vocal loudness.
    True
    False

15. Giral are most prone to develop vocal nodules.
    True
    False

16. A polyp is a benign neoplasm.
    True
    False

17. Voice therapy may involve psychological counseling skills.
    True
    False

18. Surgical treatment may completely eliminate a voice problem.
    True
    False

19. A person with a voice disorder should be seen (or have been seen) by a physician.
    True
    False

20. Voice therapy may involve increasing vocal loudness.
    True
    False

21. Voice building is a simple short process.
    True
    False

22. Neoplasms of the vocal folds may cause the voice to sound "breathy."
    True
    False

23. Hypernasality may be a congenital problem.
    True
    False

24. An artificial larynx may generate sound with pulmonary air pressure.
    True
    False

25. Following trauma, a stent can support thelaryngeal cartilages while they heal.
    True
    False

Multiple Choice

1. Poor or unplesant voice quality is called:
    a. dysphonia
    b. telephonia
    c. carcinoma
    d. aphonia

2. A sliding change in pitch without audible break is called a:
    a. vibrato
    b. glissando
    c. glycerine
    d. tremolo

3. Edema lowers vocal pitch by:
    a. increasing tension
    b. iicreasing mass
    c. increasing subglottic pressure
    d. all of the above

4. Aphonia may be caused by:
    a. disease
    b. psychological factors
    c. paralysis
    d. all of the above

5. What condition causes incomlete glottal closure through stiffening of te crocoarytenid joint?
    a. anemia
    b. paralysis
    c. conversion reaction
    d. anklyosis

6. Mass lesions of the vocal folds produce which of the following changes?
    a. alter their shape
    b. decrease their mass
    c. increase their mobility
    d. place them in the paramedian position

7. Which of the following is a malignant neoplasm?
    a. polyp
    b. cyst
    c. nodule
    d. squamous cell carcinoma

8. Which condition can cause a voice disorder?
    a. poor posture
    b. lack of exercise
    c. nasal twang
    d. anemia

9. Isolation of a specific muscle group for relaxation is a technique of...
   a. meditation
   b. differential relaxation
   c. progressive relaxation
   d. biofeedback

10. What term describes a surgically built tunnel connection the traches and the esophagus?
    a. shunt (fistula)
    b. funnel (venturi)
    c. chimney (tube)
    d. window (fenestra)

11. At what point on the vocal fold margins do nodules usually form?
    a. unilaterally at the cartilaginous portion of the folds
    b. at the anterior juncture of the folds
    c. bilaterally, in the midpoint of the membranous portion of the folds o
    d. bilaterally, at the midpoint of the vocal folds

12. Which of the followong can create edema in the vocal folds?
    a. pregnancy
    b. allergic reactions
    c. vocal abuse
    d. all of the above

13. What is the most common age for papillomata to form?
    a. six months to one year
    b. one ear to two years
    c. four years to six years
    d. eight years to fifteen years

14. Which of the following may cause a laryngeal web?
    a. surgery
    b. injury
    c. congenital factors
    d. all of the above

15. Most resonance disorders may be characterized by...
    a. breathiness
    b. nasal twang
    c. hyper- or hypo-nasality
    d. aphonia

16. What is the most ubiquitous electrical aid to voice diagnosis?
    a. a laryngeal mirror
    b. a sound recorder
    c. a sound spectrograph
    d. a boom box

17. Which childhood personality is associated with vocal abuse?
    a. shy, quiet, iterested in board games
    b. musically gifted, amiable, interested in pleasing the teacher
    c. dull, listless, interested in clothes
    d. competitive, aggressive, interested in sports

18. Which of the following is part of madical intervention in voice therapy?
    a. hyperventilation
    b. relaxation
    c. finding optimum pitch
    d. Psychiatry

19. Which of the folowing is part of direct intervention in voice therapy?
    a. Psychiatry
    b. avoiding polluting atmospheres
    c. regulation of breathing
    d. creation of a P-E segment

20. Which of the following is part of an environmental approach to therapy
    a. reducing the amount of yelling and singing
    b. excision of the nodules
    c. relaxation
    d. voice training

21. What is the physical relationship of the trachea to the esophagus?
    a. the trachea is posterior to the esophagus
    b. the trachea is anterior to the esophagus
    c. the trachea is lateral to the esophagus
    d. the trachea is inferior to the esophagus

Chapter Nine Students' Guide

The Fluency Disorder of Stuttering

Peter R. Ramig and George H. Shames

Chapter Overview

Fluency disorders are quite complex, having multiple neuromuscular and psychological sources, manifestations and cultural implications. Even among scholars and scientists who study the disorder, there is a lively discussion about causes and treatments. Normal speech contains interruptions that are hardly noticed by speaker or listener. These normal dysfluencies are differentiated from disordered fluency and cluttering. Stuttering, by whatever definition, seems to decrease under certain conditions and to increase under others. It affects more males than females, and most cases start early in life. Assessment and treatment approaches depend on the clinician's theoretical grounding and on the characteristics of a particular case.

Student Outcomes

After reading this chapter students should be able to do the following:

☞ Differentiate between STUTTERING, CLUTTERING, and NORMAL DYSFLUENCY.

☞ Describe the major theories on the development and maintenance of stuttering behavior.

☞ Detail the development of STUTTERING BEHAVIOR.

☞ Describe ASSESSMENT and INTERVENTION PROCEDURES in disorders of fluency.

☞ Identify and discuss current issues related to stuttering behaviors.

☞ Discus potential WARNING SIGNALS that alert clinicians to possible disorders of fluency.

Section:

(No Name for This Section)

Concept:

Stuttering has public and private faces. Its public face is one of involuntary interruptions in the flow of speech, while its effects on the feelings of the speaker are private. Other disorders disrupt speech, but these differ from stuttering. It can be difficult to tell normal interruptions in speech from disordered ones. Stuttering has been associated with neurological disease, but is also seen in individuals with otherwise normal nervous systems. Its severity seems to increase as anxiety increases.

1. What is the relationship of listener feelings to the identification of a fluency disorder?

2. Describe two differences between *stuttering* and *cluttering*.

    A.

    B.

3. What is the approximate incidence of stuttering in the United States?

4. What are some reasons that incidences might appear different in other countries?

5.   At what time of life does stuttering usually start?

6.   Why should a person who stutters have emotional problems?

Section:

Definition

Concept

There are several definitions of stuttering, depending on the theoretical point of view of the definer. For the purposes of this chapter, the author uses the definition put forth by Harold Wingate.

1.   List the three components of Wingte's definition of stuttering.

        A.

        B.

        C.

2.   Describe these three observable speech manifestations of stuttering:

        A.   Repetitions:

        B.   Blocks:

C.   Prolongations:

3.   What are some *secondary behaviors* associated with stuttering?

4.   What *covert behaviors* may be seen in stuttering?

Section:

Examples of Some Phenomena Associated with Stuttering

Concept:

Certain conditions seem to favor the onset of stuttering and to increase or decrease its severity. Further, most stutterers share certain genetic similarities.

1.   List nine *fluency-enhancing* conditions.

A.

B.

C.

D.

E.

F.

G.

H.

I.

2.   List four conditions that seem to be fluency-reducing.

A.

B.

C.

D.

3.   What are three reasons for the high male:female stuttering incidence ratio?

A.

B.

C.

4.   What is significant about twin studies in stuttering incidence?

5.   Give a neurological and an emotional explanation for the developmental timing of stuttering behavior.

   A.   Neurological:

   B.   Emotional:

6.   Give a genetic reason and a psychological reason for stuttering to "run in families."

   A.   Genetic Reason:

   B.   Psychological Reason:

Section:

Theories of Causation

Concept:

Theories of stuttering causation range from biological to environmental.

1.   When did Orton and Travis first put forth their theory of cerebral hemisphere competition as a source of stuttering?

2.   Why is there renewed interest in the cerebral dominance theory today?

3.   What two body systems are implicated in biochemical and physiological theories?

       A.

       B.

4.   Why do researchers posit a genetic factor in stuttering?

5.   What is the general thrust of the neuropsycholinguistic approach to stuttering causation?

6.   Name the two hypothetical components of Perkins' *et.al.* (1991) fluent speech production system.

       A.

       B.

7.   What did Postma and Kolk posit that happens when a stutterer detects a "false error"?

8.   What have scientists concluded from new imaging technology studies of neurophysiologic brain functin breakdown during stuttering.

9.　　What is meant by "diagnosogenic-semantogenic"?

10.　　What has been the general effect of psychoanalysis or traditional psychotherapy on stuttering?

11.　　In systematic desensitization therapy, what does a stutter learn to compete with his anxiety about talking?

12.　　What are Brutten and Shoemaker's two factors?

　　A.　　Classically Conditioned Factor:

　　B.　　Operantly Conditioned Factor:

13.　　What evidence supports operant conditioning as one of the factors of stuttering causation?

　　A.　　Flanagan, Goldiamond and Azrin (1958):

　　B.　　Shames and Sherrick (1963):

Section:

Multicultural Influence on Persons Who Stutter

Concept:

Recent research has found differences in the attitudes of cultures other than Anglo-Saxon on fluency.

1.   Why do researchers suppose African-American people who stutter attempt to hide and mask their stuttering?

2.   Which countries reported more cases of stuttering?

3.   Which countries reported fewer cases of stuttering?

Section:

Normal Dysfluency

Concept:

Developmental dysfluency is an aspect of normal speech development, usually observed at two and one half to three years of age.

1.   What does the author mean by *effortless* repetitions of words and syllables, and why is that different than stuttering?

Section:

The Development of Stuttering

Concept:

Most cases of stuttering appears to follow a predictable track. Beginning with the normal dysfluencies of early childhood and evolving into dysfluency associated with fear, anxiety and avoidance.

1.   List the four stages of stuttering development described by Bloodstein in 1960.

   A.

   B.

   C.

   D.

2.   Describe Van Riper's three critical stages in stuttering development.

   A.   Primary Stuttering:

   B.   Transitional Stage:

   C.   Secondary Stuttering:

3.   What are the six characteristics that differentiated Van Riper's four tracks of stuttering development?

   A.

B.

C.

D.

Section:

The Assessment Process

Concept:

The choice of an assessment procedure varies with the problems of the person who stutters and with the theoretical viewpoint of the clinician.

1.   What two clinical entities are crucial in the assessment of stuttering?

A.

B.

2.   How did Adams (1980) specify normal dysfluency?

3.   List Curlee's seven criteria that are definitive of a stuttering problem.

      A.

      B.

      C.

      D.

      E.

      F.

      G.

4.   List Ramig's (1994) nine danger signs of incipient stuttering behavior and tell why they might forecast the onset of stuttering.

      A.

      B.

C.

D.

E.

F.

G.

H.

I.

5.   For the each of the following clinical questions, indicate whether it focuses in *antecedent events, forms of speech responses,* or *consequent events.*

A.   "What was the occasion for your child's dysfluency?"

B.   "What was going on just before the stuttering?"

C.　"How often do these circumstances occur?"

D.　"What did you observe?"

E.　"Does it always look like that or does it vary?

F.　"What do you do when this happens?"

G.　"What, in general, seems to happen as a result of your child's speech behavior?"

6.　What are the advantages and disadvantages of direct observation of stuttering behavior?

A.　Advantages:

B.　Disadvantages:

7.   Name three quantitative baseline measures that are useful in the assessment of stuttering.

    A.

    B.

    C.

8.   What are three questions a clinician might ask to begin to understand the impact of stuttering in a client's life?

    A.

    B.

    C.

9.   How might the clinician's theoretical point of view bias the information gathered in an interview?

10.   What are some of the treatment choices for young children?

11.   What prognostic issues might concern a client?

Section:

Therapy for Stuttering

Concept:

Therapy approaches for stuttering are influenced by theoretical foundations of the nature and causes of stuttering. Three major schools of thought include fluency shaping, modification, and integration of shaping and modification. Variation within a given approach depends upon the age of the client. Treatment in the earlier years has been most successful.

1.   List seven approaches to stuttering therapy with preschoolers.

    A.

    B.

    C.

    D.

    E.

    F.

    G.

2.   Pick three of the sixteen influential home stuttering variables and describe how each might precipitate stuttering.

3.   Describe three approaches to psychological therapy for the young stutterer.

      A.

      B.

      C.

4.   General goals of stuttering therapy include (see text): changing *talk*; changing *feelings*; and changing *interaction*. For each of the following approaches to advanced stuttering, indicate toward which change(s) it is oriented.

      A.   Antiavoidance or Modification Therapy:

      B.   Anxiety Reduction Therapy:

      C.   Fluency-Shaping Therapy:

      D.   Feedback Therapy:

      E.   Stutter-Free Speech Enhancement

5.   Why is improvement of interpersonal relationships an important aspect of stuttering therapy?

6.   What does the author consider therapy that does not include transfer activities?

7.   Describe four activities that may enhance therapeutic transfer.

   A.

   B.

   C.

   D.

8.   What does the author mean when he posits that a stutterer can speak without stuttering before therapy?

9.   What is the difference between maintenance and relapse?

10.   What are three plausible reasons for relapse?

   A.

   B.

C.

Section:

Prevention

Concept:

Prevention of stuttering is difficult without a clear view of its causation. Part of the answer is modifying parent behavior.

1.   What are two purposes of parental counseling in the arrest of budding stuttering?

A.

B.

Section:

Final Thoughts

Concept:

Stuttering is an elusive speech disorder. Clinicians need a logical basis by which they can explain variations and similarities among stutterers.

1.   Describe the author's three proposed logics to reconcile stuttering variabilities.

    A.

    B.

    C.

Critical Terms

Define the following terms, using your text as a reference:

o   Fluency

o   DYSFLUENCY

o   Cluttering

o   Fluency Enhancing Conditions

o   Inhibition

o   Primary Stuttering

o   Secondary Stuttering

o   Maintenance

o   Fluency Shaping

o   Normal DYSFLUENCY

o   Block

o   Antecedent Event

o   Classical Conditioning

o   Developmental DYSFLUENCY

o   Prognosis

o   Baseline

o   Punishment

o   Relapse

o   Delayed Auditory Feedback

- Circumlocution

- Desensitization

- Transfer

- Prevention

- Time Pressure

Chapter Nine Self Test

True/False

1. Stuttering is simply a matter of repetitions of whole and part words.
   True
   False

2. There appears to be no familial pattern in stuttering behavior
   True
   False

3. The listener plays a role in the determination of whether or not dysfluency is a disorder.
   True
   False

4. Most cases of stuttering start in the preschool years.
   True
   False

5. The longer a stuttering problem exists, the more likely it is that associated emotional problems will develop.
   True
   False

6. People who stutter may find that whispering reduces their symptoms.
   True
   False

7. Monozygotic twins show a smaller percentage of stuttering in both children.
   True
   False

8. Stuttering and cluttering are two names for the same disorder.
   True
   False

9. Stutterers may experience greater difficulties when telling jokes.
   True
   False

10. Recent evidence has largely refuted cerebral dominance theories of stuttering causation.
    True
    False

11. There is little doubt that stuttering runs in families.
    True
    False

12. At least some overt stuttering behavior as been controlled empirically by operant conditioning.
    True
    False

13. Parents should view dysfluency in children between two and one half and three and one half years of age with great alarm.

        True

        False

14. Stuttering intervention begun at an early age has a good success record.

        True

        False

15. Visible muscular tension while speaking is a normal sign.

        True

        False

16. The most valid and reliable assessment procedures are based on direct observation

        True

        False

17. Fluency shaping involves modification of stuttering moments.

        True

        False

18. Boys who stutter outnumber girls who stutter by a ratio of 4:1.

        True

        False

19. Stuttering therapy for preschool children may involve direct intervention.

        True

        False

20. Wingate defined stuttering to include the presence of emotional states.

        True

        False

21. Systematic desensitization teaches the stutterer to do something that competes with his anxiety about speaking.

        True

        False

22. Success in treatment means no relapses.

        True

        False

23. Counseling appears to be a necessary component of the total clinical management of stuttering.

        True

        False

24. Systematic desensitization is a technique based on the orientation that stuttering is conditioned.

        True

        False

25. Experimentation has revealed that stuttering can be prevented.

        True

        False

Multiple Choice

1. Which of the following is *NOT* one of Wingate's components of stuttering?
    a. presence of emotion
    b. disruptions of speech fluency
    c. accessory struggle and tension
    d. syntactic reversals
2. Which of the following characterize people who clutter?
    a. precocious language development
    b. incomplete utterances
    c. echolalia
    d. circumlocution
3. Which of the following did Goldman (1967) report regarding cultural differences in stuttering?
    a. More females stutter than males
    b. Japanese Americans have a low incidence of stuttering when they speak English.
    c. Twice as many African American males stutter as do African American Females.
    d. British Americans place more speaking anxiety on their children.
4. Which of the following is an overt symptom of stuttering?
    a. repetitions
    b. absence of sound
    c. prolongations of sounds
    d. all of the above
5. Which of the following conditions may reduce the severity of stuttering?
    a. singing
    b. talking on the telephone
    c. telling a joke
    d. speaking to authority figures
6. According to surveys, which child is most likely to stutter?
    a. a monozygotic male twin who's twin brother stutters and who has a family history of stuttering
    b. a child with delayed language onset
    c. a child with poor dentition who speaks two languages
    d. an African American male
7. Which cerebral hemisphere to proponents of the "Cerebral Dominance" theory of stuttering causation posit is dominant?
    a. left
    b. right
    c. both
    d. neither

8. "Neurotic" theories suggest that...
      a. stuttering is a well-integrated, purposeful defense against some threatening idea.
      b. whispering is a way to hide a stutterer's emotions.
      c. the telephone is protection from direct contact with others.
      d. most young children exhibit dysfluent speech.

9. The one true cause of stuttering is...
      a. lack of cerebral dominance
      b. conditioned behavior
      c. neurophysiologic breakdown
      d. unknown

10. According to Sheehan's "approach-avoidance" construct, people who stutter have their anxieties reduced by..
      a. remaining silent
      b. speaking
      c. either speaking or remaining silent
      d. stuttering

11. According to a survey by Bloodstein (1995) regarding incidence of stuttering in different countries, in which group did the United States fall?
      a. countries with substantially less stuttering
      b. countries with an average amount of stuttering
      c. countries with substantially more stuttering
      d. countries with no stuttering

12. Which of the following statements best characterizes a child in Bloodstein's stuttering developmental "Phase 2"?
      a. occasional repetitions of initial words or syllables, little reaction
      b. chronic stutterer at times of excitement but doesn't care
      c. occasionally reacts to stuttering with irritation
      d. stuttering regarded with fearful anticipation

13. According to Curlee and Van Riper how many dysfluencies constitute stuttering?
      a. repetitions in 1% of words uttered
      b. any prolongations and hesitations in 1% of words uttered
      c. prolongations longer than one second on 2% or more of words uttered
      d. all of the above

14. According to Ramig (1990) which of the following is/are considered to be warning signals for a child exhibiting dysfluent speech?
      a. imprecise speech articulation
      b. avoidance of speech
      c. self talk during play
      d. jargon early in speech development

15. Which is the goal of "Fluency-Shaping"therapy?
    a. inhibit anxiety with counter conditioned relaxation
    b. establish left cerebral hemisphere dominance
    c. teach acceptance of the problem
    d. demonstrate ways to increase fluency and replace stuttering

16. What kind of therapy model does "Reciprocal Inhibition" fit?
    a. fluency shaping
    b. modification therapy
    c. parental training
    d. delayed auditory feedback

17. Which of the following is a fluency-shaping treatment?
    a. changing parent-child interactions
    b. psychological therapy
    c. delayed auditory feedback
    d. reciprocal inhibition

18. Researchers (Yaruss and Conture, 1995) have suggested that a parent may be speaking to fast if his/her rate of speech is...
    a. faster than that of the child
    b. two syllables per second faster than that of the child.
    c. ten syllables per second faster than that of the child
    d. it depends on the language spoken by parent and child

19. Which of the following was a therapy approach of old?
    a. putting stones in the mouth
    b. oral surgery
    c. waving one hand in the air
    d. all of the above

20. Which of the following do all therapy approaches for advanced stutterers have in common?
    a. self hypnosis
    b. focus on machinery
    c. imagery
    d. changing quality of interpersonal relationships

21. Which of the following is maintenance activity?
    a. reinforcement by family and friends for fluency in non-clinical speech activities
    b. self-rating
    c. behavioral contracting
    d. all of the above

22. Which is a necessary component of total clinical case management in stuttering?
    a. fluency-shaping
    b. metronome conditioned speech
    c. counseling
    d. delayed auditory feedback

23. Continued emission of target behaviors established during therapy is called...
    a. maintenance
    b. counseling
    c. fluency-shaping
    d. reciprocal inhibition
24. What has research demonstrated about prevention of stuttering?
    a. Prevention depends on the severity of stuttering.
    b. Prevention of stuttering has not been demonstrated empirically.
    c. Stuttering is the most preventable speech disorder
    d. One out of ten children who stutter could have been prevented from doing so.
25. Variations in treatment are partly functions of...
    a. a random choice
    b. the parents' ability to pay
    c. theoretical definition and perception of the problem
    d. ASHA recommendations

Chapter Ten Students' Guide

Hearing and Hearing Disorders

Fredrick N. Martin and Bart Noble

Chapter Summary

The perception of sound is an integral part of communication by speech. Thus, audiologists and speech pathologists share a common interest in the study of hearing and the effects of hearing disorders on the breakdown of human communication. Both professions study acoustics and how human use sound energy as language. Hearing disorders may develop before, during and after birth and affect communication to varying extent. They can involve the outer, middle and inner ear, and can affect the mechanical transmission of acoustic energy to the inner ear or the neurological functions that make the brain sort out and derive meaning from sounds. Audiologists have special tests by which they can assess hearing function and recommend therapies to accommodate hearing loss.

Student Outcomes

After reading this chapter students should be able to do the following:

☞ Discuss the prevalence of hearing disorders in the general population.

☞ Outline the major anatomical and physiological features of the auditory mechanism.

☞ Discuss the PRENATAL, PERINATAL, and POSTNATAL causes of hearing loss.

☞ Describe the effects of hearing loss on communication.

☞ Outline audiological assessment techniques

☞ Discuss various approaches for the management of hearing loss.

Critical Concepts

Section:

Introduction

Concept:

Human beings use organs of eating, drinking and breathing to encode language symbols in the form of vibrations in the air around us. These vibrations are propagated to the ear, which allows the brain to decode the symbols. Interference with the signal can occur at any point from the brain of the speaker to the brain of the listener.

1. Describe the "Speech Chain" as put forth by Denes and Pinson (1963) from the thought of the speaker to the thought of thelistener at each of the following points.

    A. Output Side:

        i. Linguistic Encoding:

        ii. Articulation and Phonation:

    B. Input Side:

        i. Peripheral Hearing Apparatus:

        ii. Reception Areas of the Brain:

2. Which professionals act in concert to remediate degradations in the fidelity of an acoustic message?

3.   Which professionals collaborate in the management of damage in the acoustic message decoding centers of the brain?

Section:

The Nature of Sound

Concept:

Sound is physically a series of pushing together and springing apart of air molecules. Acoustic physicists study certain measurements of the pushing and springing, including the distance of the push and spring, the number of times they occur in a second, and how many different pushes and springs occur simultaneously.

1.   What do physicists call the *maximum displacement* of a molecule in sound propagation?

2.   What do physicists call the *force* produced by pushing the miolecule?

3.   What do physicists call the number of times the pushing is repeated every second?

4.   Whose name is associated with *intensity*?

5.   Whose name is associated with *frequency*?

6.   What is the difference between a pure tone and a complex tone?

7.   From an acoustic viewpoint, what kind of sound is *speech*?

8.   Which speech sounds provide most of the energy (intensity) of speech?

9.   Which apeech sounds provide most of the information (intelligibility) in speech?

10.   What is prosody and how does it influence perception of speech?

Section:

Disorders of Hearing

Concept:

Disorders of hearing may affect the outer, middle and inner divisions of the ear, the auditory nerve, and the brain. The age of onset at each site may be before, during or after birth.

1.   Describe the general progression of an acoustic signal from the environment to the brain.

Section:

The Outer Ear

Concept:

The outer ear's function is to conduct sound to the tymapnic membrane and help the listener identify the location of a sound source. Damage to the outer ear causes little damage to hearing.

1.   What are the parts of the outer ear?

2.   How is the pinna bypassed by most audiological testing?

Section:

Prenatal Causes of Hearing Loss in the Outer Ear

Concept:

The greater the exposure of the individual to the environment, the greater are the number of risks to the outer ear. Exceptions to this are a number of congenital or familial differences that affect the developing embryo.

1.   What are some causes of outer ear atresia?

Section:

Perinatal Causes of Hearing Loss in the Outer Ear

Concept:

Perinatal causes of outer ear damage are mechanical.

1.   How might the outer ear be damaged during delivery?

Section:

Postnatal Causes of Hearing Loss in the Outer Ear

Concept:

Damage to the outer ear after birth my be caused by hostile environment, trauma or disease. The effects on hearing depend upon the extent of the damage. Blockages of the external auditory canal by cerumen or deliberate placement absorbs some of the sound energy before it can reach the middle ear.

1.   How would the following postnatal outer conditions affect hearing?

    A.   Burns or Frostbite:

    B.   Cancer:

    C.   Trauma (*Hint: see paragraph on trauma to the tympanic membrane)*:

    D.   Impacted Cerumen:

E.   Insertion of Foreign Objects:

F.   Infections:

G.   Tumor:

Section:

The Middle Ear

Concept:

The middle ear is a complex structure which serves to amplify the acoustic energy reaching the inner ear. Normally, its only connection to the environmental air is by means of a tube connecting it to the upper pharynx. Hearing loss associated with middle ear function is caused by compromise of its mechanical efficiency.

1.   How does the Eusachian tube allow replenishment of air in the middle ear? Why is replenisment necessary?

2.   Describe the two ways that the midle ear matches the acoustic impedance of the environment with that of the inner ear.

A.

B.

Section:

Prenatal Causes of Hearing Loss in the Middle Ear

Concept:

Prenatal causes of middle ear dysfunction may be familial predisposition or abnormal development in the womb.

1.   Differentiate the terms *genetic* and *congenital (Hint: you shuld look the terms up in a medical dictionary).*

Section:

Perinatal Causes of Hearing Loss in the Middle Ear

Concept:

Damage to the middle ear during delivery is realtively unusual.

1.   Describe how the middle ear might conceivably be damaged during delivery.

Section:

Postnatal Causes of Hearing Loss in the Middle Ear

Concept:

Otitis media is one of the most comon causes of hearing loss related to any part of the ear. It affects middle ear function through the accumulation of fluid in the tympanic cavity. Other postnatal middle ear disorders result from disease or trauma.

1.   What are three ways that infctious organisms gain acces tothe tympanic space?

   A.

   B.

   C.

2.   Why would the fluid in the middle ear afect its function?

3.   How is Otitis Media managed today?

4.   Describe an individual most likely to develop otosclerosis.

Section:

The Inner Ear

Concept:

The tiny, fluid-filled inner ear has two sections: one for balance; one for hearing. The hearing part changes the machanical energy delivered by the midle ear to electro-chemical energy that can be used by the brain.

Section:

Prenatal Causes of Hearing Loss in the Inner Ear

Concept:

Prenatal inner ear disorders include genetic syndromes, oxygen deprivation, and maternal disease. Some genetically transmitted inner ear hearing disorders diseases do not become apparent until after birth.

1.   Name two infectious diseases that may affect development of the inner ear.

    A.

    B.

2.   How migt hearing loss be associated with mental retardation or cerebral palsy?

Section:

Perinatal Causes of Hearing Loss in the Inner Ear

Concept:

The birth process can be damaging to the inner ear. There is a movement to have all babies screened at birth to identify hearing disorders as early as possible.

Section:

Postnatal Causes of Hearing Loss in the Inner Ear

Concept:

Hearing losses that develop from factors encountered after birth are called "acquired" or "adventitious." Common causes are disease and noise exposure.

1.   Name three diseases that may cause hearing loss after birth.

   A.

   B.

   C.

2.   Which artery carries blood to the inner ear?

3.   When is hearing loss asociated with age expected?

Section:

The Auditory Nerve and the Brain

Concept:

Damage to the nerve that carries sound generated neural impulses to the brain usually results in a person having dificulty with complex sounds like speech. Sometimes there is no change in the listener's responses to pure tones, leading some to think there is no hearing problem.

1.   How does the brain provide redundancy in its auditory neural pathways?

2.   What are some difficult listening situations for a person with retrocochlear damage?

Section:

Prenatal Causes of Hearing Loss in the Auditory Nerve and the Brain

Concept:

Many of the causes of prenatal coclear damage affect retrocochlear structures as well.

1.   Name three prenatal factors that can cause hearing loss in the auditory nerve and the brain.

A.

B.

C.

Section:

Perinatal Causes of Hearing Loss in the Auditory Nerve and the Brain

Concept:

Many of the causes of preinatal cochlear damage also affect retrocochlear structures.

1.   How is the brain damaged by the birth process?

Section:

Postnatal Causes of Hearing Loss in the Auditory Nerve and the Brain

Concept:

Diseases and trauma that cause damage to the brain may affect those parts that are concerned with hearing.

1.   What is the usual effect or surgical removal of a tumor from the auditory nerve?

2.   Describe the audiologist's role in the medical imaging process.

Section:

The Measurement of Hearing

Concept:

Audiological evaluation has evolved with the development of sophisticated equpiment to control test stimuli and detect responses. An essential aspect of audiological testing involves the patient's subjective responses.

1.   What does "OdB HL" mean?

2.   What is a disavantage of pure tone audiometry?

3.   Under what circumstances would an audiologist logically waive bone conduction testing without fear of losing information?

4.   If bone conduction thresholds are normal and air conduction thresholds are eleveted, what might an audiologist logically conclude?

5.   What is the normal range for air or bone conduction thresholds?

6.   Describe the three fofrms of acoustic immittance testing/

        A.   Static Immittance:

        B.   Tympanometry:

        C.   Acoustic Reflex Testng:

7.   Describe three types of tympanograms put forth by Jerger (1970).

        A.   Type A:

B.   Type B:

C.   Type C:

8.   What does the Auditory Brain-Stem Response Technique tell the audiologist?

9.   How wuld "EOAE" testing be useful with neonates?

Section:

Types of Hearing Loss

Concept:

There are four categories of hearing loss: conductive, sensorineural, mixed and central. Various types of audiolgical testing help determine the presence and extent of each type.

1.   List the three rules of audiogram interpretation.

A.

B.

C.

2.   What is the difference between a "conductive" and a "sensorineural" hearing loss?

3.   What does the author mean when he refers to the "sensory" and the "neural" part of the ear?

Section:

Implications of Hearing Loss

Concept:

Type and degree of hearing loss and age of onset are the principal determinants of the effects of a hearing loss. Of the three types, a conductive loss appears to be the least detrimental and most amenable to change. The earlier in life a hearing loss occurrs, the greater is its potential to affect the individual's lifestyle. This is particularly true before speech has developed.

1.   What is the estimated incidence of profound hearing loss among infants?

2.   How early should a child receive a hearing test?

3.   Why are postlinguistic hearing losses less detrimental?

4.   Why should an audiologist consider gestational age instead of chronological age when testing infants?

Section:

Remediation

Concept:

Hearing loss may be treated medically, surgically and by habilitation/rehabilitation.

1.   How can the communiction specialist determine how much information to present at a counseling session?

2.   Why might it be a good idea to have parents observe their child'sresponses to audiological testing?

3.   Describe the following types of hearing aids.

   A.   Body:

   B.   BTE:

   C.   ITE:

   D.   ITC:

   E.   CIC:

   F.   Eyeglass:

4.   What are the four components of all hearing aids?
   A.

   B.

   C.

D.

5. Why do hearing aid designers seek to alter the amplification characteristics of their circutry?

6. What important point must a recipient of a cochlear implant understand?

7. Why would a patient need an auditory brainstem implant instead of a cochlear implant?

8. What is the purpose of a temporal bone stimulator?

9. How does a vibrotactile aid make a person aware of sound?

10. Describe three devices that help hearing impaired people use the telephone.

A.

B.

C.

11. What is the purpose of an "ALD"?

12. List five functions for which a hearing impaired person might use an alerting device.

A.

B.

C.

D.

E.

13. List the seven components of an auditory rehabilitation program

A.

B.

C.

D.

E.

F.

G.

14. What choices in educational services do parents of deaf children have?

A.

B.

C.

D.

E.

F.

G.

15. What is the underlying assumption of the oral approach?

16. In what ways do the Deaf function in a bilingual culture?

Critical Terms

Define the following terms, using your text as a reference:

o   Speech Chain

o   Amplitude

o   Intensity

o   Sound Pressure Level

o   Sensation Level

o   Frequency

o   Pure Tone

o   Fundamental Frequency

o   Allophone

o   Auricle

o   Tympanic Membrane

o   Cerumen

o   Ossicles

o   Otitis Media

o   Secretory Otitis Media

o   Minimum AuditoryDeprivation

o   Myringotomy

o   Pressure Equalizing Tubes

o   Otosclerosis

- o   Endolymph Fluid

- o   Perilymph Fluid

- o   Cochlea

- o   Anoxia

- o   Rubella

- o   Cytomegalovirus

- o   Meniere's Disease

- o   Presbycusis

- o   Auditory Thresholds

- o   Pure Tone Average

- o   Speech Recognition Threshold

- o   Speech Detection Threshold

- o   Word Recognition (Discrimination)

- o   Audiogram

- o   Speech Banana

- o   Air Conduction

- o   Bone Conduction

- o   Acoustic Immittance

- o   Conductive Hearing Loss

- o   Sensorineural Hearing Loss

- o   Retrocochlear Hearing Loss

o   Signal Nose Ratio

o   Hearing Impairment

o   Hearing Handicap

o   Habilitation

o   Rehabilitation

o   Pre- and Post-Linguistic

o   Speechreading

o   Cued Speech

o   Total Communicaton

o   Sign Supported Speech

o   Bi-Bi

o   ASL

Chapter Six Self Test

True/False

1. Sound waves travel in all directions from the source.
    True
    False
2. Amplitude is the number of compressions and rarefactions in a given time.
    True
    False
3. The amount of particle displacement is amplitude.
    True
    False
4. Frequency is measured in Hertz.
    True
    False
5. The decibel scale is named after Alexander Graham Bell.
    True
    False
6. Most natural sounds are pure tones.
    True
    False
7. The fundamental frequency of vowels in a speech wave is the frequency of the speaker's Glottic cycle (vocal fold vibration).
    True
    False
8. The first and second formants usually provide enough information to make vowels intelligible.
    True
    False
9. Impaired perception of prosodic spec elements may result in *deaf speech*.
    True
    False
10. Most disorders of the outer ear cause significant hearing loss.
    True
    False
11. Only the mother's ingestion of drugs can affect the unborn child.
    True
    False

12. The middle ear plays a crucial role in sound localization.
> True
> False

13. The ossiclces are structures of the inner ear.
> True
> False

14. The inner ear serves two biological functions..
> True
> False

15. The *ear drum* is the entire middle ear.
> True
> False

16. Speech discrimination is measured with an SRT.
> True
> False

17. Some genetically based hearing disorders are not visible until later in life.
> True
> False

18. Hearing threshold refers to the softest sound which can be perceived 100% of the time.
> True
> False

19. ASL has the same syntax as General American English.
> True
> False

20. Pure tone audiometry results are always reliable.
> True
> False

21. An ABR is a form of hearing test.
> True
> False

22. The tympanogram measures thresholds for pure tones.
> True
> False

23. Implants may be placed directly into the brain stem.
> True
> False

24. For most people, a sound of about 85 dB SL l. will elicit a stapedial reflex.
> True
> False

25. Research suggested that deaf children who are fluent in ASL and English show superior achievement.

       True

       False

Multiple Choice

1. A crayon inserted in the external ear canal can result in what type of hearing loss?
   a. conductive
   b. sensorineural
   c. mixed
   d. central

2. ANSI established normal hearing level thresholds for pure tones at:
   a. 0 dB SL HL
   b. 50 dB SL SPL
   c. variable, depending on the tone frequency.
   d. measured electronically

3. Audiologists refer to the area of an audiogram within which most speech frequencies and intensities are located as the...
   a. sensorineural zone
   b. talking area
   c. speech banana
   d. speech fruit cocktail

4. Pure tone audiometry assesses...
   a. the type of hearing loss
   b. stapedial reflex
   c. middle ear function
   d. speech discrimination

5. Normal pure tone hearing thresholds are in what range?
   a. 0-5 dB SL HL
   b. 10-15 dB SL HL
   c. 0-10%
   d. IV-V dB SL re:.0002 dynes/cm^3

6. What happens to middle ear impedance when there is fluid in the tympanum?
   a. It increases.
   b. It decreases.
   c. It remains unchanged.
   d. It drains the fluid from the tympanic cavity.

7. Which type of tympanogram is normal in Jerger's (1970) nomenclature?
   a. Type A
   b. Type B
   c. Type C
   d. Type D

8. Which of the following factors are chief determinants of hearing loss implications for an individual
   a. age of onset
   b. type of loss
   c. degree of loss
   d. all of the above

9. What disease causes growth of bone in the oval window?
   a. measles
   b. endolymph
   c. cerebral palsy
   d. otosclerosis

10. What causes atresia of the external ear canal?
    a. trauma
    b. otitis media
    c. gestation problems
    d. ossicular discontinuity

11. A postnatal cause of hearing loss due to damage in the inner ear is:
    a. atresia
    b. otitis media
    c. rubeola
    d. all of the above

12. Pure tone audiometry...
    a. uses involuntary responses
    b. uses voluntary responses
    c. is passive
    d. uses tuning forks

13. A person with a high frequency hearing loss would encounter the greatest difficulty perceiving:
    a. /a/
    b. /s/
    c. /e/
    d. /m/

14. Zero decibels "Hearing Level" means...
    a. there is no sound.
    b. the intensity at which normal hearers can barely hear the sound.
    c. the listener has a hearing impairment.
    d. the frequency is neutral.

15. In sensorineural hearing loss, what is the usual comparison between air and bone conduction thresholds?
    a. Air conduction thresholds are lower than bone conduction thresholds.
    b. Air conduction thresholds are higher than bone conduction thresholds.
    c. Air conduction thresholds are within 10 dB SL of bone conduction thresholds.
    d. There are no bone conduction thresholds.

16. If a hearing loss occurs before the development of language it is said to be a:
    a. prelinguistic loss
    b. postlinguistic loss
    c. both of the above
    d. neither of the above

17. Which of the following is a *prosthesis?*
    a. hearing aid
    b. dental caps
    c. temporal bone stimulators
    d. all of the above

18. Which type of hearing lossis most readily curable?
    a. sensorineural
    b. cochlear
    c. conductive
    d. none of the above

19. A sound made up of multiple frequencies is said to be...
    a. complex
    b. pure
    c. complicated
    d. central

20. Infection of the middle ear is called...
    a. Meniere's disease
    b. Presbycusis
    c. Otitis externa
    d. Otitis media

21. How are neonates in medical distress identified?
    a. tattooing
    b. placement on the waiting list
    c. placement on the high-risk registry
    d. they are wrapped in purple p.j.'s

22. What is the most common complaint patients have about their hearing?
    a. They feel dizzy.
    b. They have difficulty hearing speech.
    c. They hear ringing in their ears.
    d. They have difficulty speaking.

23. What stimuli comprise most word recognition lists?
    a. sentences
    b. multisyllabic words
    c. bisyllabic words
    d. monosyllabic word

24. How long after stimulus presentation do auditory brainstem responses occur?
    a. within the first ten milliseconds
    b. after ten seconds
    c. not until one second has passed
    d. when the patient raises his/her hand

25. Which of the following is a type of hearing aid?
    a. AGC
    b. CIC
    c. ASL
    d. dB

Chapter Eleven Students' Guide

Cleft Palate

Betty Jane McWilliams and Mary Anne Witzel

Chapter Summary

Between the sixth and twelfth weeks of fetal gestation, the left and right sides of the face and facial skeleton fuse in the middle. When they fail to do so, the result is a craniofacial cleft. Various types and of clefts may occur as isolated phenomena or as part of a syndrome. Since clefts involve the anatomy of the vocal tract, varying effects on speech are predictable. However, there may be other attendant problems, including language delay, family dysfunction and self image degradation. Habilitation programs combine the efforts of specialists from several disciplines, modern diagnostic equipment and advanced surgical reconstruction techniques help the person with a craniofacial cleft assume a normal life.

Student Outcomes

After reading this chapter students should be able to do the following:

☞   Discuss prevalence and classification of clefts.

☞   Describe factors which influence the postnatal development of a child with a cleft palate.

☞   Provide an overview of speech and language characteristics of children with clefts of the palate associated with velopharyngeal incompetence and/or other dental problems.

☞   Describe techniques for assessing speech in children with cleft's and craniofacial abnormalities.

☞   Describe the interdisciplinary management of children with clefts.

Critical Concepts

Section

Introduction

Concept:

A cleft is an opening that usually results when parts arising from either side of the developing embryo fail to grow toward one another and attach in the midline of the body. In the skull, such parts include the upper lip and palate.

1.   Approximately when n fetal development do the parts of the lip and palate fuse?

2.   What is a *syndrome*?

3.   Distinguish between a *cleft lip, cleft palate,* and a *craniofacial abnormality.*

Section:

Classification of Clefts

Concept:

Clefts may occur in several patterns, depending upon which embryonic structures fail to fuse. Several systems of cleft classification enable specialists to plan treatment and communicate with one another. The most useful system is an anatomical description of the laterality end extent of the opening.

1.   Describe the following types of orofacial clefts:

   A.   Left unilateral complete:

   B.   Bilateral complete:

   C.   Isolated palatal cleft:

   D.   Unilateral (left) cleft lip:

   E.   Submucous cleft:

2.   What are the features that provide clues to the possibility of a submucous cleft?

Section:

Other Structural or Functional Abnormalities

Concept:

Abnormal dimensions of the oropharynx and nasopharynx or motor coordination of their musculature may complicate the problems of palatal clefts.

1.   What dimensions of the pharynx might further compromise the ability of an abnormal velum to close the velopharyngeal sphincter?

2.   What role might a neurologist play in the diagnosis and treatment of velopharyngeal incompetence?

Section:

Craniofacial Abnormalities

Concept:

Craniofacial abnormalities are structural defects of the head and face. These defects may be part of a syndrome that includes other abnormalities. Consequences include structural and developmental anomalies.

1.   Why might language development be delayed in a child with a craniofacial abnormality?

Section:

Prevalence

Concept:

Clefts appear to vary in occurrence among different populations.

1.   Why is incidence information useful for the speech-language pathologist?

2.   From the information given in the text, describe the race and gender of an individual most likely to have a cleft.

Section:

Underlying Mechanisms

Concept:

Clefts are most likely to be caused by multiple factors, including genetic predisposition and detrimental environment. Some clefts, however are the result of genetic factors only.

1.   How can a parent's behavior cause an unfavorable environment for a fetus?

2.   What is a *genetic* cause?

3.   How should a genetic counselor use racial incidence information in working with patients?

Section:

Diagnosis

Concept:

Speech-language pathologists must assess. the interaction of several interacting factors that have the potential to affect communication in the person with a cleft. Among these factors are feeding, hearing, and development of psychosocial, mental, language and speech articulation skills.

1.   Why do babies with clefts have difficulty feeding?

2.   Describe possible strategies of the speech-language pathologist in counseling parents about feeding their babies who have clefts.

     A.   Verbal and Tactile Communication with the Feeding Infant:

     B.   Nipple Design and Feeding Position:

3.   How does the speech-language pathologist help manage hearing in children with clefts.

4. Why is there less risk for hearing impairment in children who have clefts of the lip only?

5. What are the speech-language pathologist's main concerns about psychosocial development in children with clefts?

6. What do recent findings suggest about mental development in children with clefts?

7. What conditions might children with clefts be at risk for delayed mental development?

8. Why might speech development be slow in children with clefts?

9.   Which speakers might have persistent articulation problems even after the cleft has been repaired and velopharyngeal competence is adequate?

Section:

Diagnostic Procedures

Concept:

Speech-language pathologists must be competent listeners above all to determine which of the many avenues should be explored in the evaluation of communication in people with clefts. The clinician applies these listening skills to rate the patient's speech acceptability as well as its intelligibility. These may be satisfactory following successful surgery. For patient's with residual speech problems, areas of special concern include language development, control of the nasal airway and resonance during speech, compensatory muscular actions, and phonatory disorders.

1.   What is turbulence?

2.   Describe how a speech-language pathologist uses a mirror in the evaluation of speech. *(Hint: Practice this yourself!)*

3.   Why do some speaker's with clefts grimace when they speak?

4.   How does the speech-language pathologist determine *nasality*?

5.   To which phonemes should a speech-language pathologist listen when listening for hyponasality?

6.   What is the *cul-de-sac resonance* test?

7.   Give four sources of articulation disorders in people with clefts.

      A.

      B.

      C.

      D.

8.   What phoneme is most likely to elicit nasal air escape?

9.   Describe four compensatory articulatory strategies seen in people with clefts.

      A.

      B.

      C.

D.

10. Why might a speaker with a cleft have to learn new phonological rules?

11. What are three signs of phonatory stress heard in some speakers with clefts?

    A.

    B.

    C.

12. What kinds of phonatory disorders might follow such stresses?

13. Distinguish between *intelligibility* and *acceptability*.

Section:

Diagnostic Tools and Methods

Concept:

Diagnostic instruments include articulation tests and devices to allow velopharyngeal function and nasal resonance to be observed in the clinic. There are some clinical methods that may indicate resonance or airflow problems, but these are no substitute for more accurate diagnosis with modern equipment.

1.   What articulation test does the author r recommend and why?

2.   Since the velopharyngeal sphincter is not easily visible on oral inspection, why do speech-language pathologists perform oral examinations?

3.   Describe the following methods in the assessment of velopharyngeal valving:

   A.   Air-pressure and Flow Techniques:

   B.   Nasometry:

   C.   Radiological Techniques:

      I.   Cephalometry:

      ii.   Cinefluoroscopy:

iii.   Videofluoroscopy:

D.   Nasendoscopy:

4.   What are five advantages of multiview videofluoroscopy?

A.

B.

C.

D.

E.

5.   List four advantages and five disadvantages of nasendoscopy.

A.   Advantages:

I.

ii.

iii.

iv.

B.

I.

ii.

iii.

iv.

v.

Section:

Treatment Approaches

Concept:

Speech problems caused by anatomical deformities are not readily amenable to speech therapy. Surgical and orthodontic methods may improve function of the speech mechanism, but it cannot operate beyond its structural limitations. Speech therapy may be helpful in teaching the client to correct inefficient movement patterns, variant phonology or other language deficits.

1. Describe the goal of the pharyngeal flap operation:

2. What other surgical technique may improve velopharyngeal valving?

3. Why should orthodontic treatment begin before speech therapy?

4. Give rationales for beginning articulation therapy before completion of a pharyngeal flap operation and for waiting until after the operation is completed.

   A. "Therapy should begin *before* the operation."

   B. "Therapy should wait until *after* the operation."

5.   How does the speech-language pathologist determine which phonemes should respond best to therapy?

6.   Under what circumstances might articulation therapy improve velopharyngeal function?

Critical Terms

Define the following terms, using your text as a reference:

o   Cleft

o   Syndrome

o   Bilateral Complete Cleft

o   Isolated Palatal Cleft

o   Submucous Cleft Palate

o   Velopharyngeal Valve

o   Nasal Escape

o   Turbulence

o   Nasalance

o   Facial Grimace

o   Hypernasality

o   Cul-De-Sac Resonance

o   Oral-Nasal Fistula

o   Hypo-Hypernasality

o   Rugae

o   Maxillary Arch Collapse

o   Buccal Sulcus

o   Tensor Veli Palatini

o   Nasendoscopy

o   Multiview Videofluoroscopy

o   Nasometry

o   Pharyngeal Flap Operation

o   Prosthetic Speech Aid

Chapter Eleven Self Test

True/False

1. Structures of the face and palate fuse between the sixth and twelfth weeks of gestation.
   - True
   - False
2. A perceptive parent can encourage communication better than a certified speech-language pathologist.
   - True
   - False
3. All oral clefts are easily detected by visual inspection.
   - True
   - False
4. Several researchers have described a "Cleft Palate Personality."
   - True
   - False
5. Most infants with palatal clefts also have middle ear pathology..
   - True
   - False
6. Most children with complete clefts are also mentally retarded.
   - True
   - False
7. Males are more likely to have clefts than are females.
   - True
   - False
8. Orientals have a higher incidence of clefts than Blacks.
   - True
   - False
9. A cleft palate cannot occur without a cleft of the lip.
   - True
   - False
10. Syndromes of congenital malformations are phenotypic expressions of genotypic traits.
    - True
    - False
11. Articulation secondary to velopharyngeal incompetence are the ones we worry about most.
    - True
    - False

12. Negative intraoral air pressure is required for normal nursing.
    True
    False
13. The tensor veli palatini muscles play a partial role in eustachian tube function.
    True
    False
14. Success of initial surgery is usually doubtful.
    True
    False
15. Children with clefts talk more than other children.
    True
    False
16. Language differences in children with clefts are less marked at later ages.
    True
    False
17. Visible nasal air escape is observed with a mirror.
    True
    False
18. When a speaker tries to valve with the nostrils, the result is a facial grimace
    True
    False
19. Hypernasality is the likely result of enlarged adenoids.
    True
    False
20. An opening from the palate into the nose is called an oral-nasal fistula
    True
    False
21. The sibilants are most affected by velopharyngeal incompetence.
    True
    False
22. A high narrow palate with excessive maxillary tissue is likely to be present in Apert's syndrome.
    True
    False
23. Surgical correction of the velopharyngeal valve will eliminate articulation errors.
    True
    False
24. Nasometry reveals nasal air flow problems.
    True
    False

25.   A prosthodontist specially designs speech aids for the individual patient.
                   True
                   False

Multiple **Choice**

1.   What kind of vocal tract resonance results when an anteriorly blocked nasal cavity is
       coupled with the rest of the vocal tract?
                   a.   hyponasal
                   b.   hypernasal
                   c.   hypo-hyper nasal
                   d.   cul de sac
2.   A submucous cleft is...
                   a.   easily observed with a mirror
                   b.   caused by trauma to the roof of the mouth
                   c.   a true muscular cleft
                   d.   isolated in the upper lip
3.   Which of the following groups have the highest incidence of clefts?
                   a.   females
                   b.   Blacks
                   c.   Caucasians
                   d.   Orientals
4.   What term describes defects of the head and face.
                   a.   Teratology
                   b.   Craniofacial abnormalities
                   d.   Syndactyly
                   e.   Esophoria
5.   Which of the following techniques can help a baby with a cleft nurse successfully?
                   a.   placing the baby in a supine position
                   b.   early switching to a cup
                   c.   holding the baby upright
                   d.   feeding with the baby in a prone position
6.   Which of the following may be the basis for speech articulation problems in children with
       clefts.
                   a.   maturational lags
                   b.   dental anomalies
                   c.   hearing loss
                   d.   all of the above

7. If the dental arch is involved in a cleft, how is the cleft classified?
   a. isolated
   b. complete
   c. submucous
   d. lip

8. Which phonemes are most likely to be produced with some nasal air escape?
   a. vowels
   b. glides
   c. fricatives
   d. plosives

9. What speech characteristic is most commonly associated with velopharyngeal incompetence?:
   a. cul de sac resonance
   b. hypernasality
   c. hyponasality
   d. denasality

10. Which articulatory compensatory posture is common among speakers with clefts?
    a. lisping
    b. labialization
    c. tongue backing
    d. tongue fronting

11. What phonatory behavior is thought to cause vocal problems among people with clefts?
    a. retention of subglottic air
    b. using too high a vocal pitch
    c. loud speech
    d. speaking on supplemental air

12. What are the medical therapies for middle-ear disease?
    a. aeration tubes
    b. myringotomy
    c. antibiotics
    d. all of the above

13. Which visualization technique is the most inclusive?
    a. cephalometry
    b. cinefluoroscopy
    c. multiview videofluoroscopy
    d. nasendoscopy

14. One estimate of the prevalence of cleft disorders in the black population ranges from:
    a. 1 in 3000 births
    b. 1 in 500 births
    c. 1 in 750 births
    d. 1 in 1200 births

15. Which surgical procedure is used to improve velopharyngeal valving?
    a. tracheostomy
    b. myringotomy
    c. tonsillectomy/adenoidectomy
    d. pharyngeal flap

16. Which professional creates dental appliances?
    a. Orthodontist
    b. Prosthodontist
    c. Dentist
    d. Velodontist

17. The least invasive articulation disorder attributable to velopharyngeal incompetence is:
    a. reduced intraoral pressure on sibilants
    b. reduced intraoral pressure on plosives
    c. glottal stops
    d. pharyngeal fricatives

18. An opening from the palate into the nasal cavity is called a...
    a. cranial fossa
    b. pharyngotympanic tube
    c. oral-nasal fistula
    d. bifid uvula

19. Nasal semivowel production is likely to be distorted when the speaker is...
    a. hyponasal
    b. hypernasal
    c. aphasic
    d. dysphagic

20. The nasometer measures
    a. turbulence
    b. nasal air emission
    c. velopharyngeal insufficiency
    d nasal resonance

21. What can multiview videofluoroscopy show?
    a. presence or absence of an opening between the oral and nasal cavities during speech
    b. an estimate about the size of the opening
    c. the shape of the orifice
    d. all of the above

22. Which is a disadvantage of nasendoscopy?
    a. it is expensive
    b. it is invasive
    c. it does not involve radiation
    d. it can be used by a speech pathology aide

23. What is an alternative surgical treatment to pharyngeal flap?
    a. implant
    b. laryngeal flap
    c. lingual frenum section
    d. prosthesis
24. After surgical treatment, gross articulatory errors are treated with...
    a. prosthesis
    b. speech therapy
    c. orthodontia
    d. no treatment is required
25. When should correction of major dental anomalies should take place?
    a. before speech therapy
    b. during speech therapy
    c. after speech therapy
    d. the timing is not crucial

Chapter Twelve Students' Guide

Neurogenic Disorders of Speech

Leonard La Pointe, Richard C. Katz and James C. Hardy

Chapter Summary

Neurogenic disorders of communication result from malformation, disease or injury to the peripheral or central nervous systems. Although the term *neurogenic* suggests an array of disorders, including those with cognitive, affective and linguistic attributes, this chapter limits the discussion to the motor speech disorders of dysarthria and apraxia. Dysarthria and apraxia are speech disorders that inhibit the integrated and rhythmic muscular functions required for speech. This inhibition can take the several forms, depending upon what part of the complex nervous system is affected. Careful assessment involves analysis of the interactions of the speech system components. Satisfactory treatment involves instruction and demonstration of strategies to maximize residual function in the context of the patient's communicative needs, and counseling to assist the patient's accommodation, motivation and understanding.

Student Outcomes

After reading this chapter, students should be able to do the following:

☞   Define terminology related to motor speech disorders.

☞   Differentiate between characteristics associated with DYSARTHRIA and APRAXIA OF SPEECH.

☞   Identify the major variables that can influence movement patterns.

☞   Identify the 7 major structures involved in the generating or valving of the speech air stream.

☞   Discuss the CAUSES and PREVALENCE of motor speech disorders.

☞   Discuss assessment and intervention procedures specific to motor speech disorders.

☞   Discuss the POINT-PLACE MODEL for evaluation of the functional components of the motor speech system.

Critical Concepts:

Section:

Classifications and Definitions

Concept:

The neurogenic communication disorders that are the focus of this chapter are output transmissive disorders such as apraxia and several types of dysarthria.

1.   List ten terms used to label neurogenic speech disorders.

      A.

      B.

      C.

      D.

      E.

      F.

      G.

      H.

      I.

      J.

Section:

Dysarthria

Concept:

Dysarthria affects speech through disruption of muscular motion and synchrony in several speech system components.

1.   List Darley, Aronson and Brown's (1975) five motor speech process.

   A.

   B.

   C.

   D.

   E.

2.   What are the movement functions of the nervous system?

   A.

   B.

   C.

   D.

   E.

3.   Differentiate the authors' *negative* and *positive* dysfunctions of dysarthria.

    A.   Negative Functions:

    B.   Positive Functions:

Section:

Apraxia

Concept:

Apraxia is a neurogenic impairment in the capacity to purposefully control the production speech. It is not a paralysis.

1.   Using Table 12.2, distinguish the symptoms of *dysarthria* from those of *apraxia* in the following areas.

    A.   Articulatory Accuracy:

    B.   Substitution Errors:

    C.   Initiation of Speech:

D.   Articulation of Consonant Clusters:

E.   Groping:

F.   Consistency of Production Quality:

Section:

Basic Concepts

Concept:

The motoric impairment of dysarthria and apraxia is fundamentally a disruption of normal movement. An understanding of the control variables underlying normal movement enhances a clinician's insight and effectiveness in treatment of conditions in which control may be disrupted.

1.   Describe how each of the following control variables described by Netsell (1986) may impair range, velocity or direction of speech movements.

      A.   Strength:

B.   Tone:

C.   Timing:

2.   Why do you think factors such as fatigue or fear can interfere with speech movements?

Section:

Components of the Motor Speech System

Concept:

The "Point Place" is a framework for analyzing the motor speech system in terms of seven coordinated muscle groups. Although the normal execution of speech movements requires concerted interaction of all the groups, such a framework can facilitate diagnosis and treatment of motor speech disorders.

1.   List the seven muscular "valves" or "generators" of the motor speech system.

A.

B.

C.

D.

E.

F.

G.

Concept:

Causes of Neurogenic Speech Disorders

Concept:

Any condition that can affect the human nervous system can disrupt normal speech movement.

1. List seven causes of neurogenic dysfunction to which communication disorders may be secondary diagnoses. Begin with the most common cause.

    A.

    B.

    C.

    D.

    E.

F.

G.

2.   Why do you think that African American people may be more susceptible to stroke than people of other races?

Section:

Characteristics and Types

Concept:

Motor disorders of speech vary widely. Their type and severity depend on the location and extent of nervous system damage.

Section:

Dysarthria

Concept:

Motor disorders affect two main aspects of speech: intelligibility and "bizarreness." They do this by disrupting the smooth interactions necessary for creation of the segmental and surpasegmental aspects of speech.

1.   What are the four characteristics in the authors' clinical checklist and how may they affect intelligibility or bizarreness?

      A.

B.

C.

D.

2.   Why is *bizarreness* an important target for clinical intervention?
Section:

Clusters of Deviant Speech Dimensions

Concept:

Darley, Aronson and Brown (1975) described five types of dysarthria. The differentiation of these types has have become fundamental to the diagnostic process.

1.   List the five types of dysarthria described by Darley, Aronson and Brown (1975) and describe their salient features.

A.

B.

C.

D.

E.

2.   If type and severity of dysarthria are dependent upon the location and extent of nervous system damage, how do you think a *mixed* dysarthria might occur?

Section:

Apraxia of Speech

Concept:

Voluntary execution of complex, patterned movements, including speech, requires formulation of a program of movements. Apraxia is impairment of the ability to realize these planned movements and may exist apart from linguistic disorders and dysarthrias.

1.   List the three cardinal features of apraxia.

        A.

        B.

        C.

2.   What role do you think the sensations of touch and sound play in formulating movement patterns?

3.   How might patterning play a role in the following rare disorders?

   A.   Palilalia:

   B.   Echolalia:

   C.   Pseudo Foreign Accent:

   D.   Aprosodia:

Section:

Assessment

Concept:

The evaluation process in a hospital or rehabilitation unit usually begins with delivery of a "Request for Services" form. This form contains a brief sketch of the patient's recent medical history. Its then up to the clinician to visit the patient and fill in the answers to the questions, "What's wrong?" and, "What should I attempt to correct?"

1.   List seven purposes of evaluation for neurogenic speech disorders.

   A.

B.

C.

D.

E.

F.

G.

Section:

Evaluation Strategies

Concept:

Lacking standardized, commercially available tests for assessing motor speech disorders, the speech-language pathologist arrives at a diagnostic starting point by sampling patient responses in four areas.

1.   What *personal history* items should be of interest to the speech-language pathologist?

2.   What *nonspeech movements* may relate to speech movements?

3.   What are the four stages of swallowing?

      A.

      B.

      C.

      D.

4.   Why is it important to observe conversational speech?

5.   List special speech tasks at each point-place "valve along the Nile."

    A.   Respiration:

        I.   *Pressure and Endurance*:

        ii.   *Quick control:*

    B.   Phonation:

    C.   Resonance:

    D.   Articulation:

6.   Why is it important to observe imitative movements when assessing apraxia of speech?

7.   Why would the following signs suggest developmental *apraxia* instead of a phonological disorder?

       A.   Increasing error count as utterances get longer.

       B.   Presence of oral apraxia.

       C.   Groping postures of speech muscles.

       D.   Prominence of voicing errors.

Section:

Interpretation and Findings

Concept:

One of the most important skills of the speech pathologist is that of deriving a diagnostic conclusion from observations of patient behavior. These conclusions include considerations of outcome and benefit in treatment planning.

1.   What is the most important consideration where multiple speech problems exist?

Section:

Treatment

Concept:

Advances in clinical management of neurogenic communicative disorders have provided hope where there was once despair. Five basic principles provide a foundation for treatment as the clinician guides the patient from drill to daily communication needs, sometimes acting in concert with other professionals.

1.   List the five principles of treatment in motor speech disorders.

     A.

     B.

     C.

     D.

     E.

2.   Describe ways the clinician can gain knowledge of treatment results.

3.   How can the clinician manipulate session organization to enhance patient benefit?

Section:

Specific Treatment Goals

Concept:

Development and statement of specific treatment goals are essential to effective care planning. Eight suggested goals may apply to dysarthria, apraxia or both. These goals should be modified to suit the particular case.

1.   Provide a *quantifiable* objective for each of the eight goals below.

    A.   Help the Patient Become a Productive Person.

    B.   Modify Posture, Tone and Strength of Speech Musculature.

    C.   Modify Respiration.

    D.   Modify Phonation.

E.   Modify Speech Resonance.

F.   Modify Speech Articulation.

G.   Modify Prosody.

H.   Provide an Alternative Communicative Mode

Section:

Counseling

Concept:

Counseling is an important part of the service provided by the speech-language pathologist. Effective counseling can augment therapeutic effects by educating the patient, increasing motivation and modifying environmental factors.

1.   What information might a patient require regarding motor speech disorders?

2.   Why might a patient *not* want to return to normal communicative abilities?

Critical Terms

o   Central Nervous System

o   Peripheral Nervous System

o   Neurogenic

o   Dysarthria

o   Apraxia of Speech

o   Strength

o   Tone

o   Timing

o   Flaccid Dysarthria

o   Spastic Dysarthria

o   Ataxic Dysarthria

o   Swallowing

o   Hyperkinetic Dysarthria

o   Hypokinetic Dysarthria

o   Prosody

o   Non-speech Movement

301

o   Point-Place System

o   CVA

o   Drill

o   Task Continua

o   Behavioral Context

o   Hyperadduction

o   Hypoadduction

Chapter One Self Test

True/False

1. More brain area is devoted to control of the speech musculature than for the lower extremities.
    True
    False

2. Dysarthria of speech refers to difficulty to formulate spoken language units.
    True
    False

3. Neurogenic speech disorders can be caused by neoplasms.
    True
    False

4. Race or ethnic factors play no role in nervous system damage.
    True
    False

5. A good short term goal for modification of respiration is producing a pressure of 5mm of water for five sec.
    True
    False

6. Sometimes braces of slings can increase the firmness of the speech production system's foundation.
    True
    False

7. Neurogenic communication disorders may affect the spinal or cranial nerves of the peripheral nervous system.
    True
    False

8. Speech movement depends solely on muscular strength.
    True
    False

9. Articulatory accuracy in volitional speech is more difficult for the patient with apraxia.
    True
    False

10. Firearms-related injury is the leading cause of head trauma.
    True
    False

11. Dysphagia is always accompanied by dysarthria of speech.
    True
    False

12. The first thing a clinician must decide is what type of dysarthria is present.
    True
    False

13. The patient with dysarthria frequently gropes for an articulatory target.
    True
    False

14. Patients with dysarthria usually have no difficulty initiating speech.
    True
    False

15. Approximately one in five Americans has some kind of neurological or communication disorder
    True
    False

16. The most prevalent cause of neurotoxicity is alcohol and drug abuse.
    True
    False

17. Lesions located in small critical brain areas can produce severe impairment.
    True
    False

18. Apraxia can affect the execution of non-speech movements.
    True
    False

19. Therapeutic goals for modifying prosody are only appropriate for patients with apraxia.
    True
    False

20. Hypokinetic dysarthria is a result of Parkinson's disease
    True
    False

21. Traumatic brain injuries affect more people over forty years of age than it does any other age group.
    True
    False

22. Speech-language pathologists are concerned only with speech intelligibility.
    True
    False

23. Spastic dysarthria is associated with brainstem disorders.
    True
    False

24. Disorders of multiple motor systems can result in mixtures of several dysarthria types.
    True
    False

25. Experience will enable the clinician to classify dysarthria type in any case.
                 True
                 False

Multiple Choice

1. Which of the following is a neurogenic communication disorder?
    a. oral apraxia
    b. literal paraphasia
    c. dysarthria
    d. all of the above

2. Speech intelligibility is negatively influenced by...
    a. involuntary movements
    b. inadequate range of movement
    c. excessive rate
    d. uninhibited activity of intact nervous system parts

3. Which of the following is a characteristic of apraxia?
    a. frequent substitution errors
    b. simplification of consonant clusters
    c. consistent quality of production
    d. no difficulty in speech initiation

4. What term describes the relatively constant state of muscular contraction?
    a. strength
    b. timing
    c. organization
    d. tone

5. Which of the seven point-places affects prosody?
    a. 1
    b. 2
    c. 4 -7
    d. all

6. What is the principle feature of resonance that a clinician assesses?
    a. harshness
    b. pharyngeal tension
    c. oral-nasal resonance balance
    d. oral-buccal resonance

7. Motor impairment of which speech system components most affects intelligibility?
    a. articulatory
    b. respiratory
    c. resonance
    d. phonatory

8.   Which dimensions of speech are affected by dysarthria?
          a.   content and relevance
          b.   intelligibility and bizarreness
          c   syntax and phonology
          d.   pragmatics and initiation

9.   Which of the following may be a cause of neurogenic speech disorders?
          a.   trauma
          b.   cerebral palsy
          c.   snake bites
          d.   all of the above

10.   The term *flaccid dysarthria* is associated with:
          a.   marked hypotonicity
          b.   marked hypertonicity
          c.   marked tremor
          d.   none of the above

11.   Ataxia is a disorder of:
          a.   the cerebral cortex
          b.   the brainstem
          c.   the peripheral nervous system
          d.   the cerebellum

12.   Variability of production patterns is a characteristic of ...
          a.   apraxia
          b.   ataxia
          c.   hypokinetic dysarthria
          d.   spastic dysarthria

13.   The Point-Place System assesses valves in which direction?
          a.   superior to inferior
          b.   lateral to medial
          c.   central to peripheral
          d.   inferior to superior

14.   If a native language speaking patient has a foreign accent, it may be a sign of...
          a.   pseudoforeign accent
          b.   pseudobulbar palsy
          c.   pseudomonas bacillus
          d.   pseudolinguistic prosodius

15.   A child who demonstrates increased errors as utterance length increases may have what disorder?
          a.   dysarthria
          b.   aphasia
          c.   developmental apraxia
          d.   phonological disorder

16. What is the first question the assessing clinician must answer?
    a. does a significant problem exist?
    b. what is the nature of the impairment?
    c. how handicapping is the condition?
    d. are some language functions intact?

17. What activity does integral stimulation treatment involve?
    a. modification of sitting posture
    b. deriving one phonetic posture from another, similar one
    c. modeling of speech postures
    d. application of surface electrodes to the fixed articulator.

18. Which of the following long-term objectives applies when return to minimal speech function is not possible?
    a. train in use of artificial larynx
    b. return to normal speech function
    c. train in resonance modification
    d. train in use of alternative communicative device

19. "Tapping" might be an activity in what kind treatment?
    a. modification of phonation
    b. modification of resonance
    c. modification of articulation
    d. modification of prosody

20. The purpose of counseling with patients who have neurogenic communicative disorders in includes...
    a. conveyance of information
    b. provision of emotional support
    c. improve environmental communication variables
    d. all of the above

21. The development of progressively more difficult speech tasks involves what strategy?
    a. developing task continua
    b. drill
    c. the points along the Nile
    d. Ethel Merman therapy

22. Which type of therapy requires the consultation of other professionals?
    a. modification of respiration for speech
    b. modification of posture
    c. modification of articulation
    d. modification of prosody

Chapter Thirteen Students' Guide

Aphasia and Related Disorders

Carol S. Swindell, Audrey L. Holland and O.M. Reinmuth

Chapter Summary

Aphasia is the most prevalent adult language problem. most often occurring suddenly in life's later years, it results from damage to parts of the cerebral hemispheres that control language processes. Cerebral hemisphere damage may be of varying extent and location, depending upon the mechanism of injury. Consequently, aphasia may be manifested in various ways. Further, cerebral hemisphere injury can result in disorders that are related to, but not the same as, aphasia. Children are susceptible to aphasia, with the striking differences depending upon their developmental stages and their youthful recuperative abilities. The study of aphasia has been approached in several ways, and classification, diagnosis and treatment may depend upon the clinician's theoretical background. Not only does aphasia affect the life of the patient, aphasia is a disorder that affects people in the patient's life as well as the patient, and an important part of the cliician's duties include counseling.

After reading this chapter students should be able to do the following:

☞   Describe basic nueroanatomy and brain function.

☞   Differentiate between FLUENT and NONFLUENT aphasias.

☞   Discuss the characterisitcs of aphasia related disorders.

☞   Identify the three basic types of stroke related to aphasia

☞   Discuss in detail the diagnostic procedures and intervention alternatives for the patient with aphasia.

☞   Identify the behavioral characterisitcs of persons with aphasia.

Critical Concepts

Section:

Aphasia and the Brain

Concept:

Damage to the thin outer covering of the cerebral hemispheres is the most frequent cause of aphasia. This covering, called the cerebral cortex, has regions attributed grossly with different movement, sensation and cognitive functions. Damage to one or more of these regions impairs their specific functions as well as their ability to act in concert.

1. Name two ways scientists have inferred loalization of functions in the regions of the cerebral cortex?

2. What are the shortcomings of each of these methods?

3. Damage to what cerebral region is most likely to produce aphasia?

4. How is the laterality of movement system grossly arranged in the nervous system?

5.   How has nauture been careful to protect the two most important language sensations?

6.   Describe the cognitive operations currently held to be the province of the right hemisphere?

7.   Using figure 13.2, find the region posterior to the fissure of Rolando and superior to the fissure of Sylvius. What communicative function does this region serve?

8.   How are the lobes of the cerebral cortex named?

9.   Name the lobes of the cerebral cortex and give the *gross* communication they serve.

      A.

      B.

      C.

      D.

10.   Use figure 13.2 to locate *Wernicke's area* and *Broca's area*. How does damage to each region affect communication?

      A.   Wernicke's Area:

B.   Broca's Area:

11.   Describe the general characteristics of *Fluent Aphasia* and *Nonfluent Aphasia*.

A.   Fluent Aphasia:

B.   Nonfluent Aphasia:

Section:

Syndromes of Aphasia

Concept:

Aphasic syndromes are clusters of language dysfunctions. Aphasiologists have recognized similarities in the effects of cortical damage corresponding to the regions of that damage. These similarities are important in studying the brain's function in language, but they are not invariant. Clinical manifestations may be unique to the patent, and the multidimensional point of view stresses examination of a patent's particular symptoms.

1.   Using the text and table 13.1, list the names of the fluent and the nonfluent aphasias.

A.   Fluent Aphasias:

i.

ii.

iii.

iv.

B.   Nonfluent Aphasias:

        i.

        ii.

        iii.

Section:

Mechanisms of Aphasia

Concept:

Lesions of the central nervous system affect its function by killing or otherwise inhibiting neurons. Lesions may be caused by several machanisms, including trauma, starvation, infection and mechanical pressure. The most common cause is stroke, which robs the neurons of nourishment.

1.   How does a stroke affect the functions of neurons?

2.   Name and describe the three types of strokes

        A.

        B.

        C.

3.   What distinguishes the language effects of general cerebral damage from those of more focal lesions?

Section:

The Person With Aphasia

Concept:

Key to the effective rehabilitation of aphasia is an understanding of the personality effects such a devastating condition can have. Clinicians understand that they are treating people rather than conditions.

1.   How would the inability to communicate your needs and wants compromise your self-image?

2.   What are three ways that brain damage can change the patient's cognitive proceses?

      A.

      B.

      C.

3.   List the four paramount family problems reported by Webster and Larkins (1979).

    A.

    B.

    C.

    D.

Section:

The Natural Recovery Process in Aphasia

Concept:

A certain amount of language recovery occurrs as a natural part of the healing process following injury to the central nervous system. This recovery is termed "spontaneous" and depends upon the patient's constitution, the extent of the injury and the quallity of care. Research has supported the benefit of speech therapy to optimize the aphasic patient's recovery, but there is still controversy over when therapy should begin.

1.   What period post-injury does evidence suggest is crucial for spontaneous recovery?

2.   When do YOU think therapy for aphasia should begin? Why?

Section:

The Assisted Recovery Process in Aphasia

Concept:

successful rehabilitation of patients with aphasia requires a multidisciplinary team of medical and paramedical specialists. Speech therapy consists of with evaluation and treatment according to the needs of the patient.

1.   List some members of an optimal rehabilitation team for aphasia.

2.   What is the fundamental difference between evaluation carried out soon after brain damage and that carried out later?

3.   Whatare the similiarities among the commercial tests of languae abilities?

4.   Describe the distinguishing features of the following commercial tests of language abilities.

   A.   *Boston Diagnostic Aphasia Examination*

   B.   *Porch Index of Communicative Abilities*

C.   *Communicative Ability in Daily Living*

5.   What are the major considerations involved in planning therapy for aphasia?

6.   Describe the basic philosophyunderlying the following treatment approaches.

    A.   Cortical Reorganization:

    B.   Reauditorization:

    C.   Deblocking:

    D.   Meloic Intonation Therapy:

    E.   Visual Action Therapy:

F.   Application to Learning Principles:

G.   Alternate Strategies:

H.   Promoting Aphasic Communication Effectiveness:

7.   What were the major conclusions of Wertz, *et al.* (1984a) regarding therpeutic effectiveness?

A.   Does speech therapy for aphasia help?

B.   Can therapy be carried out at home?

C.   When should therapy start?

Section:

Related Disorders

Concept:

The symptoms of acquired aphasia in children, head injury in adults and right hemisphere damage are similar to aphasia. There are diferences that among these related disorders that require special approaches to treatment.

1. Describe the differences between children and adults in the lauguage disturbances that follow cerebral injury.

   A. Symptoms:

   B. Recovery:

2. Why might the rehabilitation team for acquired aphasia in children require two speech-language specialists?

3. What are three salient features of closed head injury in adults?

   A.

   B.

C.

4. Describe the patient's behavioral characteristics and treatment implications of the following stages of the *Rancho Los Amigos Hospital's Levels of Cognitive Recovery*.

   A. *RLA 2-3:*

   B. *RLA 4-6:*

   C. *RLA 7-8+:*

5. What prominent communication changes are associated with right hemisphere damage?

Critical Terms

Define the following terms, using your text as a reference:

o   Aphasia

o   Hemiplegia

o   Hemiparesis

o   Hemianopisa

o   Unilateral Neglect

o   Hemisphere

o   Cortical

o   Subcortical

o   Lateral

o   Posterior

o   Anterior

o   Occipital Lobe

o   Parietal Lobe

o   Temporal Lobe

o   Wernicke's Aphasia

o   Fluent Aphasia

o   Broca's Aphasia

o   Nonfluent Asphasia

o   Neologistic Jargon

- o Press of Speech

- o Literal (Phonemic) Paraphasias

- o Verbal (Semantic) Paraphasias

- o Anomic Aphasia

- o Conduction Aphasia

- o Agrammatism

- o Mixed Aphasia

- o Global Aphasia

- o Stroke

- o Perseveration

- o Stereotypes

- o Agnosia

- o Apraxia

- o Spontaneous Recovery

- o Reauditorization

- o Acquired Aphasia

- o Head Injury

- o Right Hemisphere Disorders

- o ArteriovenousMalformation

- o Saccular (Berry) Aneurysm

- o Transcortical Sensory Aphasia

o   Transcortical Motor Aphasia

Chapter One Self Test

True/False

1. The most common cause of aphasia is "stroke."
   - True
   - False

2. Right hemispheres lesions can affect the way a patient uses speech prosody.
   - True
   - False

3. Self-concept may be jeopardized as a result of aphasia.
   - Tru
   - False

4. The right hemisphere contains the centers for language function in most individuals.
   - True
   - False

5. Wernicke's aphasia is on of the *nonfluent* aphasias.
   - True
   - False

6. Aphasia has been caused by damage to subcortical structures.
   - True
   - False

7. Aphasia in children is treated the same as aphasia in adults.
   - True
   - False

8. Visual impulses generated n the right eye are processed only by the left cerebral hemisphere.
   - True
   - False

9. Loss of vision in half of the visual field is called quadrantal anopsia.
   - True
   - False

10. Lesions of the right hemisphere sometimes produce unilateral *neglect*.
    - True
    - False

11. The inability to recall the names of objects is *agrammatism*.
    - True
    - False

12. Initiation of speech is generally left unimpaired in nonfluent aphasias.
    True
    False

13. Damage to Wernicke's area produces difficulties on comprehending speech.
    True
    False

14. Substitution of in-semantic-class words, such as "knife" for "fork" are called phonemic or literal paraphasias.
    True
    False

15. *Broca's aphasia* is characterized by sparse, slow, labored speech.
    True
    False

16. Some recovery from aphasia is likely to occur after a few months, with or without therapy.
    True
    False

17. The majority of studies are equivocal regarding the effectiveness of speech therapy for aphasia.
    True
    False

18. Fluent aphasias are most commonly the result of lesions in the posterior part of the dominant cerebral hemisphere.
    True
    False

19. Children with acquired aphasia rarely demonstrate any significant degree of recovery.
    True
    False

20. Formal evaluation is most useful immediately following a cerebral injury or as soon as possible.
    True
    False

21. Destruction of the visual cortex of one hemisphere would result in hemianopsia.
    True
    False

22. *Reauditorizaton* is a term that describes the reorganization of auditory processes during recovery from aphasia.
    True
    False

23. The *Porch Index of Communicative Abilities* is the only aphasia instrument that seeks to predict recovery potential.
    True
    False

24. Melodic intonation therapy is a carefully sequenced series of activities that helps the patient reestablish representational behavior through gestures.
    True
    False

25. We do not know how the brain capitalizes on therapy activities.
    True
    False

Multiple Choice

1. Most children acquire aphasia as a result of...
    a. developmental delays
    b. neonatal hypoxia
    c. head injury or diseases
    d. lack of stimulation

2. Which of the following language disturbances most often results from brain damage in the posterior speech areas?
    a. fluent speech
    b. auditory comprehension difficulties
    c. slow, labored speech
    d. motor programming deficits

3. In which aphasia pattern is almost normal language marred by word retrieval difficulties?
    a. Conduction aphasia
    b. Broca's aphasia
    c. Wernicke's aphasia
    d. Anomic aphasia

4. What type of paralysis results from damage to the motor cortex of one cerebral hemisphere?
    a. hemiplegia
    b. diplegia
    c. athetosis
    d. quadriplegia

5. Which of the following is a type of "stroke?"
    a. embolism
    b. hemorrhage
    c. thrombosis
    d. all of the above

6. If a patient presents with unilateral right hemiplegia, to which cerebral hemisphere might we infer damage?
    a. right hemisphere
    b. left hemisphere
    c. both hemispheres
    d. neither hemisphere

7. Why is any paralysis combined with aphasia most often a right hemiplegia?
    a. Aphasia most often results from damage to the left cerebral hemisphere.
    b. Hemiplegia is a language disturbance following a stroke.
    c. Hemiplegia most often involves the ipsilateral hemisphere.
    d. Strokes are the most common cause of aphasia.

8. Which of the following is not an aphasia treatment approach?
    a. Melodic Intonation Therapy
    b. Reauditorization
    c. Visual Action Therapy
    d. Neurodevelopmental Treatment

9. Which of the following is most true about aphasia?
    a. It is a speech disorder.
    b. It is a breakdown in the ability to process the symbols of language
    c. It has gradual onset.
    d. It is a learned condition

10. The use of *Stereotypes* is most associated with:
    a. Broca's aphasia
    b. Wernicke's aphasia
    c. Global aphasia
    d. Mixed aphasia

11. Interruption of blood flow through the left cerebral artery in adulthood is most likely to produce which disorder?
    a. left unilateral neglect
    b. aphasia
    c. flaccid dysarthria
    d. left hemiplegia

12. Which area of the brain is of most interest to aphasiologists?
    a. pons
    b. cortex
    c. basal ganglia
    d. corpus callosum

13. Which of the following is a *nonfluent* aphasic syndrome?
    a. Wernicke's
    b. Conduction
    c. Transcortical Sensory
    d. Global

14. One commonly-held theory about the jargon of Wernicke's aphasia supposes that...
    a. The patient has paralysis of the muscles of speech articulation.
    b. The patient has difficulty comprehending her own speech.
    c. The patent has difficulty with word retrieval.
    d. The patient has difficulty programming the muscles of speech.

15. Which of the following mechanisms is most likely to produce focal cerebral deficits?
    a. stroke
    b. closed head trauma
    c. diabetic coma
    d. anoxia

16. Which of the following is generally thought to be a *right* hemisphere function?
    a. word retrieval
    b. speech programing
    c. short term memory
    d. music appreciation

17. The chronically aphasic patient is one...
    a. who continues to improve two months post onset.
    b. for whom spontaneous recovery has reached a plateau.
    c. has had a recent exacerbation.
    d. receives no further benefit from therapy.

18. Of the following tests of aphasia, which attempts to profile aphasic syndromes?
    a. *Boston Diagnostic Aphasia Evaluation*
    b. *Western Aphasia Battery*
    c. *Communicative Ability of Daily Living*
    d. *Porch Index of Communicative Abilities*

19. Language behaviors that result from closed head trauma are:
    a. motor
    b. among generalized deficits
    c. focused on a certain language modality
    d. focal language deficits

20. On the *Rancho Los Amigos Hospital's Levels of Cognitive Recovery Scale*, which level is the closest to independence?
    a. RLA 2
    b. RLA 5
    c. RLA 6
    d. RLA8

21. How have we inferred localization of cerebral cortical functions?
    a. experimental lesions in animals
    b. direct stimulation of human subjects' brains
    c. relating post mortem findings with case history data
    d. all of the above

22. Damage to which of the following areas has the highest likelihood of producing nonfluent aphasia?
    a. Broca's area
    b. the left occipital lobe
    c. Wernicke's area
    d. the right temporal-parietal juncture

23. How long post onset in the period during which most spontaneous changes in language deficits have occurred?
    a. 24 hours
    b. one week
    c. 30 days
    d. 60 days

24. Which of the following is one purpose of all formal tests of language ability?
    a. measurement of patient's intelligence quotient
    b. disentangle the source of a patient's difficulty on a language task
    c. profile the patient's aphasic syndrome
    d. predict recovery potential

25. In Wertz', *et al.* (1984a) study of aphasia treatment effectiveness how did the group that did not receive therapy for twelve weeks perform after twelve subsequent weeks of therapy?
    a. poorer than the groups that received therapy for the whole time
    b. better than the groups that received therapy for the whole time
    c. the same as the groups that received therapy the whole time
    d. like they had never had aphasia

Chapter Fourteen Students' Guide

Augmentative and Alternative Communication

Kathleen Kangas and Lyle Lloyd

Chapter Summary

Alternative or augmentative communication (AAC) extends the communicative abilities of individuals who are unable to meet their normal communication needs through conventional speech or handwriting. AAC strategies include training individuals to optimize their residual abilities through unaided or unaided means. Through unaided means, the individual with the communicative disorder uses his or her own body to enhance communication through different modalities. Technological advances have led to the development of aided communicative means with a variety of formats and applications. The speech-language pathologist teams with other rehabilitation professionals to match the device to the needs of the person. Assessment and intervention considerations are discussed, and the chapter concludes with a section dealing with advocacy and the Public Laws as they pertain to AAC.

Student Outcomes

After reading this chapter, students should be able to do the following:

☞ Discuss ASSESSMENT and INTERVENTION considerations for the AAC client.

☞ Identify the characteristics and factors that contribute to the success of AAC.

☞ Distinguish between AIDED and UNAIDED communication devices.

☞ Compare and contrast CENTER BASED ASSESSMENT PROCEDURES with NATURALISTIC ASSESSMENT PROCEDURES.

☞ Define AUGMENTATIVE AND ALTERNATIVE COMMUNICATION.

☞ Discuss the role of the INTERDISCIPLINARY TEAM in the management of the AAC client.

Critical Concepts

Section:

Functions of AAC

Concept:

The term "Augmentative and Alternative Communication" is cumbersome, but it aptly describes the wide variety of strategies and procedures used to assist people who are otherwise unable to meet their communication needs and wants.

1.   What type of disability or disabilities might require a person to employ *Augmentative* communication?

2.   What type of disability or disabilities might require a person to employ *Alternative* communication?

Section:

Categories of AAC

Concept:

A key concept in the implementation of AAC is the understanding of the two broad categories: "Aided" and "Unaided."

1.   Describe a means of "Unaided" AAC.

2.   Describe a means of "Aided" AAC.

Concept:

AAC Model

Concept:

AAC strategies are based on a broad communication model which has six components. Strategic implementation of involves manipulation of three aspects of the AAC process according to the exigencies of the individual case.

1.   List the six components of the *AAC communication model.*

      A.

      B.

      C.

      D.

      E.

      F.

2.   List the three aspects of the *AAC process.*

      A.

      B.

      C.

3.   Give examples of two *unaided* "means to represent" and two *aided* "means to represent."

      A.   *Unaided* means to represent:

            I.

    ii.

  B.   *Aided* means to represent:

    I.

    ii.

4.   What is an advantage of a symbol *system* over a symbol *set*?

5.   What criteria should the therapist consider when considering symbol systems for a client?

6.   Give examples of two *aided* "means to select" and two *unaided* "means to select."

  A.   Aided Selection:

    I.

    ii.

  B.   Unaided Selection:

    I.

    ii.

7.   What are the important considerations involved in selecting a scanning system?

8.   Describe the following types of scanning systems.

     A.   Visual Scanning:

     B.   Auditory Scanning:

     C.   Linear Scanning:

     D.   Row-Column Scanning:

     E.   Block Scanning:

     F.   Direct Scanning:

     G.   Step Scanning:

     H.   Automatic Scanning:

9. What considerations are involved in choosing a satisfactory switch for scanning?

10. Give two examples of *unaided* "means to transmit" and two examples of *aided* "means to transmit."

    A. Unaided Transmission Means:

        I.

        ii.

    B. Aided Transmission Means:

        I.

        ii.

11. Suggest how some users of AAC might be encouraged to be multimodality communicators?

Section:

Reason for AAC success

Concept:

AAC appears to facilitate communication development in six ways. Research is needed to substantiate these and identify others.

1.   Describe how AAC facilitates communication development in the six ways below:

     A.   Simplification of Input:

     B.   Enhanced Response Production:

     C.   Advantages for Individuals with Severe Cognitive Impairment:

     D.   Receptive Language/Auditory Processing Advantages:

E.   Stimulus Processing/Stimulus Association Advantages:

F.   Symbolic Representational Advantages:

Section:

Communicative Competence

Concept:

Selection of an appropriate AAC strategy includes consideration of the prospective user's overall competence in communication. This overall competence may be viewed as inclusive of four component competencies.

1.   What are the components of *linguistic competence*?

2.   What *operational competencies* must a normal communicator demonstrate?

3. Why might an individual who needs AAC need development in the realm of *Social Competence*?

4. What are the two fundamental skills involved in *Strategic Competence*?

    A.

    B.

Section:

Potential Users of AAC

Concept:

Impairments that may cause individuals to require AAC can be congenital or acquired, and strategic exigencies may differ accordingly. Other essential considerations in planning are individual abilities in motor, cognitive and sensory domains.

1. What motor considerations are important in AAC approaches?

2. What are the shortcomings of the usual methods for determining cognitive status in those with severely limited communication abilities?

3.   What sensory channels are important to communication?

4.   Why is it important to begin AAC with very young, congenitally disabled children?

5.   What is the goal of AAC intervention for the adolescent or adult with severely limited communication functions?

6.   What kinds of *acquired* disabilities might lead to the need for AAC intervention?

7.   What is the long-range goal of AAC intervention with individuals who have acquired severe communication disabilities?

8. What kinds of strategies are most useful for temporary AAC applications?

Section:

Assessment

Concept:

Familiarity with available AAC strategies and aids enables the assessing clinician to develop a plan the for individual patient. An important additional consideration is the environments in which the client is to communicate.

1. What are three features that the clinician must match to the AAC strategy?

    A.

    B.

    C.

2. How can sensory deficits affect the success of AAC message transmission?

3. How should the clinician interpret standardized test results with people who have severe sensory or motor impairments?

4.   What role does *culture* play in the planning of AAC intervention?

5.   What are two advantages of "criteria-based" assessment over "maximal assessment" in AAC planning?

    A.

    B.

6.   What are the advantages of the *Center-Based* assessment approach?

7.   What are the advantages of the *Naturalistic Assessment* approach?

Section:

Intervention

Concept:

Intervention is based on the consensus of a team of rehabilitation specialists and the individual with the disability. The focus is on the needs and wishes of the disabled individual.

1.   Why is it important a rehabilitation teams efforts are coordinated?

2.   Name a possible long-range objective of an AAC intervention plan.

3.   Name a possible short-range objective of an AAC intervention plan.

4.   What is the role of the client's family in developing the intervention plan?

5.   How can AAC be a solution to challenging behavior in a child with severely limited communication abilities?

Section:

Funding, Rights, and User Perspectives

Concept:

Obtaining funding for AAC devices and consultation can be part of the speech-language pathologist's role. Clinician have ethical and legal responsibilities in implementing the disabled individual's civil rights through AAC or other means.

1.   Name three possible funding sources for AAC intervention.

      A.

      B.

      C.

2.   What is ASHA's standpoint on the use of AAC intervention?

3.   What public law may cover the speech-language pathologist's responsibility in AAC treatment?

4.   What are two concerns expressed by disabled individuals about the quality of intervention?

      A.

      B.

5. What are three professional organizations concerned with rehabilitation of persons with disabilities?

    A.

    B.

    C.

Critical Terms

Define the following terms, using your text as a reference:

o   Alternative Communication

o   Augmentative Communication

o   AAC

o   Aided AAC

o   Unaided AAC

o   Means to Represent

o   Means to Select

o   Means to Transmit

o   Symbol Sets

o   Ideograms

o   Symbol System

o   Iconicity

o   Perceptual Distinctness of Symbols

o   Complexity

o   Direct Selection

o   Scanning

o   Visual Scanning

o   Linear Scanning

o   Row-Column Scanning

o   Block Scanning

o   Direct Scanning

o   Step Scanning

o   Automatic Scanning

o   Digitized Speech

o   Transmission

o   Digitized Speech

o   Synthesized Speech

o   Dedicated Devices

o   Multimodal Communication

o   Strategic Competence

o   Operational Competence

o   Social Competence

o   Functional Communication

o Linguistic Competence

o Partner-Assisted Training Scanning

Chapter Fourteen Self Test

True/False

1. AAC intervention is only suitable for those who have acquired communication disorders.
   True
   False

2. AAC use might replace a reason for challenging behavior in children.
   True
   False

3. Augmentative devices are designed to communicate an entire message.
   True
   False

4. Operational competence is not important in AAC intervention.
   True
   False

5. American Indian hand talk uses a symbol system.
   True
   False

6. Iconicity has been associated with learning success in mentally retarded individuals.
   True
   False

7. Direct selection methods are those in which the possible choices are offered in sequence.
   True
   False

8. One possible aided selection technique uses eye gaze to indicate a symbol on a clear acrylic board.
   True
   False

9. In partner-assisted auditory scanning, the speakers partner speaks out the options on the array.
   True
   False

10. Infants and toddlers are too young to derive benefit from AAC.
    True
    False

11. Bliss symbols have a high degree of iconicity.
    True
    False

12. Synthesized speech systems can produce virtually any message.
    True
    False

13. Dedicated AAC devices are designed to perform functions beyond communication.
    True
    False

14. Multimodal communication includes facial posture, facial expression and gestures in addition to the spoken signal.
    True
    False

15. A weakness of AAC devices is that they have poor figure-ground differential.
    True
    False

16. Learning that a symbol represents a referent is easier when they both exist in the same stimulus mode.
    True
    False

17. Graphic symbols have the advantage of permanency
    True
    False

18. The user's sensory capabilities are important in planning AAC strategy.
    True
    False

19. Social competence varies between cultural contexts.
    True
    False

20. The clinician is well-advised to obtain funding for a dedicated electronic alternative communication device for a patient with a temporary communicative disability.
    True
    False

21. The patent who cannot move his upper extremities is not a candidate for a dedicated AAC device.
    True
    False

22. Standardized assessments are perfectly suitable for rating cognitive functions in potential AAC users.
    True
    False

23. Some AAC users may attend college classes.
    True
    False

24. Digitized speech sounds more natural that synthesized speech.
    True
    False
25. Criteria-based assessments reduce the extent of information gathered to begin a particular intervention.
    True
    False
26. The potential AAC user's family may provide important information for planning intervention.
    True
    False
27. AAC devices can be programmed applications of the user's personal computer..
    True
    False

Multiple Choice

1. Aided AAC techniques require:
    a. external equipment
    b. picture boards
    c. switching devices
    d. no external equipment
2. Which of the following is an aspect of the AAC process?
    a. means to remember
    b. means to reproduce
    c. means to represent
    d. means to relate
3. Which of the following is symbol system?
    a. American Indian Hand Talk
    b. Picsyms
    c. Lexigrams
    d. American Sign Language
4. Unaided symbol systems...
    a. require an external device.
    b. attach one meaning to one symbol.
    c. are collections of ideograms.
    d. are rule-based and expressed with the speakers body.
5. Communication devices that require external equipment are referred to as:
    a. aided devices
    b. dedicated devices
    c. unaided devices
    d. none of the above

6. Which of the following symbols has the greatest amount of *iconicity?*
    a. a printed word
    b. a line drawing of the object
    c. a spoken word
    d. a gesture

7. Which of the following statements is true regarding symbol systems?
    a. They have a greater representational range than symbol sets.
    b. They can represent abstract and concrete concepts equally well.
    c. They have their own linguistic rules.
    d. all of the above

8. Symbol complexity (in Blissymbols) is...
    a. the number of lines used to make up the symbol
    b. the number of meanings the symbol can have
    c. the degree of abstractness of the symbol
    d. the material of which the symbol is composed

9. Which of the following is a consideration for symbol selection?
    a. the cost
    b. culture of the potential speaker
    c. sensory demands
    d. all of the above

10. The degree to which symbols seem different is called:
    a. complexity
    b. iconicity
    c. perceptual distinctness
    d. all of the above

11. Which of the following concepts is concrete?
    a. love
    b. dog
    c. man
    d. hat

12. Which of the following is a characteristic thought to affect symbol learning?
    a. iconicity
    b. complexity
    c. perceptual distinctness
    d. all of the above

13. Using a head stick to point to a symbol is an example of...
    a. unaided scanning
    b. aided direct selection
    c. unaided direct selection
    d. directed selection

14. Which type of scanning is the slowest and most cumbersome?
    a. linear scanning
    b. row-column scanning
    c. block scanning
    d. directed scanning

15. The user must stop the scanning with a switch in which type of scanning?
    a. linear scanning
    b. row-column scanning
    c. block scanning
    d. automatic scanning

16. Means to transmit refers to...
    a. the manner in which the communication partner receives the message.
    b. the array of possible symbols used for communication.
    c. the type of scanning employed by the sender.
    d. how the individual chooses the symbols.

17. Which type of speech is a computer encoding phonemes through acoustic algorithms?
    a. synthesized speech
    b. digitized speech
    c. both of the above
    d. neither of the above

18. An advantage of synthesized speech is...
    a. high intelligibility
    b. low memory requirement
    c. high degree of naturalness
    d. ease in programming

19. An advantage of digitized speech is:
    a. low memory requirements
    b. great flexibility
    c. good quality signal
    d. unlimited number of possible messages

20. Adapted strategies that are called into play in the event of a communication breakdown are components of...
    a. linguistic competence.
    b. operational competence.
    c. social competence.
    d. strategic competence.

21. Social competence includes the communication skills of...:
    a. phonology
    b. sociolinguistics
    c. semantics
    d. tactical linguistics

22. A *feature matching* approach consists of...
    a. ensuring the patient will use the AAC device.
    b. matching users who have the same devices.
    c. matching therapists who share the same theoretical backgrounds.
    d. matching features of the AAC strategy or device with the needs of the client.

23. The ability of the client to comprehend the symbol system depends on which skills?
    a. cognitive and sensory
    b. dexterity and coordination
    c. social and pragmatic
    d. none of the above

24. Early use of AAC might be directed in which direction?
    a. increasing the child's self-talk
    b. increasing the child's participation in daily routines
    c. increasing the child's appreciation for electronic technology
    d. increasing the manual dexterity of the child

25. Which of the following disabilities may call for temporary use of AAC?
    a. dysarthria
    b. ALS
    c. cerebral palsy
    d. tracheostomy

26. In which assessment format is the client able to try several different AAC devices?
    a. center-based assessment
    b. maximum assessment
    c. naturalistic assessment
    d. standardized assessment

27. Examiners using commercial standardized tests in AAC assessment must remember what when interpreting results?
    a. Children become fatigued easily.
    b. The norm-references are no longer valid.
    c. Norm tables are grouped by age.
    d. Scores should be reported by using an AAC device.

28. Public law 101-336 protects...
    a. the civil rights of disabled individuals.
    b. racial hiring preferences.
    c. equal educational opportunity.
    d. the rights of clinicians in all disciplines.

Chapter Fifteen Students' Guide

Cerebral Palsy

James C. Hardy

Chapter Summary

Cerebral Palsy is a diagnostic category that describes an array of disorders, linked by the presence of damage to the nervous system structures that control movement, occurring and completed before or around the time of birth. The mechanisms that cause cerebral palsy may also affect other nervous system functions, leading to a syndrome that has manifestations and associated conditions that range from mild to severe. It is distinct from nervous system disorders that are acquired later in life because it changes the general maturation of the nervous system and, hence, may affect the individual's cognitive, communicative and social development. Habilitation of individuals with cerebral palsy is a team effort, and team members must have a thorough understanding of the modern techniques and sciences of their disciplines to determine the strengths and limitations imposed by the condition in each case.

Student Outcomes

After reading this chapter, students should be able to do the following:

☞ Define terminology and characteristics relevant to CEREBRAL PALSY

☞ Discuss characteristics speech, language, and communication disorders observed in this population

☞ Discuss the role of AUGMENTATIVE COMMUNICATION SYSTEMS for persons with cerebral palsy

☞ Discuss the importance of interdisciplinary team management with this population.

☞ Identify various assessment and intervention approaches used with people displaying developmental neuromotor disorders.

Critical Concepts

Section:

(Introduction)

Concept:

Cerebral palsy has been studied for over a century. The condition is an abnormality of the developing brain that presents an array of manifestations, with the distinguished by the presence of a nonprogressive neuromotor system dysfunction resulting from conditions present around the time of birth.

1.   What were the contributions of the following physicians to the study of cerebral palsy?

     A.   W. J. Little:

     B.   Sigmund Freud:

2.   What two characteristics are fundamental to the diagnosis of cerebral palsy?

     A.

     B.

Section:

Incidence

Concept:

Incidence statistics of cerebral palsy depend upon diagnostic approaches of different health care administration regions. The incidence is sufficiently high to support the need for special service delivery programs.

1.   What is the range of "stated" incidences of cerebral palsy given in the text?

Section:

Etiology

Concept:

Several mechanisms can damage the developing brain before or during birth. An important factor underlying the extent of damage is the time in gestation during which the determining mechanisms operate.

1.   When are neural mechanisms most susceptible to damage?

2.   How do the following mechanism affect nervous system development?

    A.   Anoxia:

    B.   Hemorrhage:

    C.   Infections:

    D.   Toxins:

E.   Trauma:

F.   Malnutrition:

G.   Prematurity:

2.   What are the two most frequent causes of cerebral palsy?

Section:

Types of Neuromotor Disorders in Cerebral Palsy

Concept:

Since the etiological factors that operate in cerebral palsy exert their influence during a period of rapid growth, their effects are more general. Thus, in cerebral palsy there are only a few variations of motor disorders.

1.   Describe the roles of the following components of general movement:

A.   Tone:

B.   Initiation and Control:

C.   Sensation:

D.   Reflex:

2.   List five types of movement disorder seen in cerebral palsy. Indicate which is the most prevalent:

A.

B.

C.

D.

E.

Section:

Abnormal Reflex Behaviors

Concept:

Reflex patterns are movement of muscles or groups of muscles which occur without conscious control of the individual. Mature reflexive behavior is the end product of refinement and inhibition of immature patterns, allowing the individual to concentrate on movement goals rather than on movement execution. Failure of the nervous system to mature normally may allow more immature reflexive patterns to interfere with smooth, directed movement.

1.   What is the difference between an *excitatory* mechanism and an *inhibitory* mechanism?

2.   Why is some degree of stretch reflex desirable in normal movement?

3.   What type of motor dysfunction is associated with too much stretch reflex?

4.   Give an example of a reflexive behavior that a normal individual can inhibit.

5.   Give an example of a helpful infantile reflex.

6.   Give an example of a reflexive behavior in very young human beings that also appears in less evolved species.

Section:

Distribution of Abnormal Muscle Function

Concept:

The effects of cerebral palsy on specific muscle groups depends upon the type and extent of the damage to the central nervous system.

1.   What is the basic difference in muscle group dysfunction between spastic and dyskinetic cerebral palsy?

2.   Which type of cerebral palsy is most likely to be associated with dysarthria of speech?

Section:

Changing Signs

Concept:

As the nervous system continues to mature after birth, the signs of cerebral palsy also change.

1.   What is the most common maturational change observed in the motor sighs associated with cerebral palsy?

Section:

Communication Disorders

Concept:

Since the distinguishing characteristic of cerebral palsy is the presence of a developmental movement disorder, the primary communication disorder associated with the condition involves difficulty moving the speech musculature.

1.   What is the relationship of mental retardation to the motor speech disorders of cerebral palsy?

Section:

The Distinguishing Characteristic: Developmental Dysarthria

Concept:

Developmental Dysarthria is distinguished from acquired dysarthria by its time of onset. the individual with developmental dysarthria has never had the experience of normal speech and requires a specialized habilitation program.

1.   What is the similarity in motor speech disorder manifestation between individuals with spastic and those with dyskinetic cerebral palsy?

2.   Why do *functional overlays* occur?

3.   What is the primary speech problem in individuals with respiratory dysfunction?

4.   What is the relationship of laryngeal, velopharyngeal and/or articulatory dysarthria to respiratory efficiency?

5.   Under what circumstances will dysarthria of the respiratory muscles leave speech intelligibly unaffected?

6.   What vocal fold movement dysfunction results in a breathy sounding voice?

7.   What vocal fold movement dysfunction results in a strained or strident sounding voice?

8.   How does velopharyngeal incompetency affect both the respiratory and the articulatory aspects of speech?

9.   Describe *differential dysfunction* of the tongue, lips and jaw.

10.   How can *dysprosody* interfere with communication in the presence of good speech intelligibility?

Section:

Other Bases of Communication Disorders

Concept:

Since cerebral palsy is caused by damage to the developing brain, the presence of problems beyond its neuromotor aspect is not surprising. Planned remediation programs must include identification of contributing factors other than the movement disorder.

1.   What is the estimated incidence of mental retardation among individuals with cerebral palsy?

2.   Why is there a higher incidence of high frequency hearing loss among individuals with cerebral palsy?

3.   What is the mos likely cause of language disorders in children with cerebral palsy?

4.   Why is it important for children to be able to demonstrate their language competence?

5.   What are current thoughts regarding the existence of developmental apraxia of speech?

6.   How do the following sensations play roles in communication development?

A.   Touch Sensation:

B.   Vision:

7.   What does the speech-language pathologist need to remember about the psychosocial effects of cerebral palsy on...

A.   the child with cerebral palsy's family:

B.   the child with cerebral palsy:

8.   Describe the three aspects of working with parents as partners in treatment of the child with cerebral palsy.

A.

B.

C.

Section:

The Necessity of an Interdisciplinary Approach

Concept:

Cerebral palsy is a complex condition that requires the consultation of professionals from several disciplines. Speech-language pathologists must know the roles of other team members in relationship to their own roles.

1.   List the essential members of a cerebral palsy team.

2.   Who are the most critical members of the team?

Section:

Systems for Improvement of Motor Function

Concept:

Although several treatment systems have been proposed to improve the muscle functions of individuals with cerebral palsy, none has been proven successful.

1.   What are the two main components of the Bobath's treatment system?

     A.

     B.

2.   What is probably the real significance of The Bobath's (neurodevelopmental treatment) program?

Section:

Postural Support Systems

Concept:

Artificially supporting a person with cerebral palsy's posture can inhibit reflexes and optimize motor performance.

1.   Name three health professionals that are consultants for constructing postural support appliances.

    A.

    B.

    C.

Section:

Remediation of Communication Disorders

Concept:

Speech-language pathologists can be most helpful to people with cerebral palsy if they understand the potentials imposed by the condition and the limitations of rehabilitation regimes.

1.   What may be the best course of action in cases where speech cannot be improved?

2.   If there is no potential for oral communication what is the next best course of action?

3.   What are the two most common limiting factors in habilitation of individuals who have cerebral palsy?

A.

B.

4.   What is the current thought regarding the relationship between speech and non-speech movements?

5.   What are the two key principles involved in increasing the effectiveness of oral communication in individuals who have cerebral palsy?
A.

B.

6.   How can a palatal lift help improve the speech of a person with cerebral palsy?

7.   What principle underlies using AAC devices with very young children who have cerebral palsy?

8.   In what two ways can parents help the child who communicates with an AAC device?

A.

B.

9.   Why might "low-tech" devices be most suitable for a person with cerebral palsy?

Section:

The Era of Assistive Technology

Concept:

Mankind has developed the technology and recognized the need to help individuals with cerebral palsy and other disorders. In the United States we have also developed a legal framework to encourage implementation of programs to achieve these ends.

1.   What was the purpose of the "Technology-Related Assistance for Persons with Disabilities Act" of 1988?

2.   What was the purpose of the "Americans with Disabilities Act" of 1990?

Critical Terms

Define the following terms, using your text as a reference:

o   Cerebral Palsy

o   Prenatal

o   Natal

o   Postnatal

o   Flaccidity

o   Embryo

o   Fetus

o   Anoxia

o   Hemorrhage

o   Bilirubin

o   Kernicterus

o   Respiratory Distress Syndrome

o   Hypertonia

o   Hypotonia

o   Hyperkinesia

o   Hypokinesia

o   Ataxia

o   Athetosis

o   Dyskinesia

o   Tension Athetosis

o   Chorea

o   Tremor

o   Spasticity

o   Reflex

o   Paraplegia

o   Diplegia

o   Quadriplegia

o   Kernicterus

o   Developmental Dysarthria

Chapter Fifteen Self Test

True/False

1. The incidence of cerebral palsy is so low that special programs are not required.
    True
    False
2. Cerebral palsy is caused only by hemorrhage in the brain
    True
    False
3. Low birth weight is a common cause of cerebral palsy.
    True
    False
4. Mental retardation rarely accompanies cerebral palsy.
    True
    False
5. A distinguishing characteristic of cerebral palsy is that it is progressive.
    True
    False
6. An estimate of the incidence of occurrence of cerebral palsy is 1.5-2 children per 1000 births.
    True
    False
7. Spasticity is the most prevalent form of neuromotor dysfunction in cerebral palsy.
    True
    False
8. Hypokinesia is not seen in cerebral palsy.
    True
    False
9. Ataxia is a neuromotor dysfunction characterized by uninhibited stretch reflex.
    True
    False
10. The term *athetosis* is being supplanted by the term *dyskinesia*.
    True
    False
11. Dyskinesia is the most prevalent neuromotor dysfunction observed in cerebral palsy.
    True
    False

12. Infants exhibit reflexive patterns similar to the movements of reptiles
        True
        False

13. Reflexes that hold our bodies upright depend, in part, upon the positions of our heads.
        True
        False

14. Spasticity is a mental condition associated with cerebral palsy.
        True
        False

15. A person with hemiplegia has paralysis of both lower extremities.
        True
        False

16. Developmental apraxia has been determined to be a frequent characteristic of cerebral palsy.
        True
        False

17. Sensations originate through activation of the central nervous system.
        True
        False

18. Dysprosody has no effect on communication efficiency.
        True
        False

19. The unique and distinguishing communication disorder of persons with cerebral palsy is dysarthria.
        True
        False

20. High frequency hearing loss is associated with damage to the developing brain.
        True
        False

21. Trauma is an infrequent cause of cerebral palsy.
        True
        False

22. For children with no potential of improving speech, dismissal from therapy is probably best for all involved.
        True
        False

23. With modern electronics, there is no longer any use for "low-tech" augmentative/alternative communication devices.
        True
        False

24   The motor disorders that accompany cerebral palsy are quite similar to those acquired by some people as adults.

        True

        False

25.   Postural support systems are of little use in cases of cerebral palsy.

        True

        False

Multiple Choice

1.   Cerebral palsy is essentially...
   - a.   a progressive neuromotor disorder.
   - b.   a progressive perceptual disorder.
   - c.   a nonprogressive intellectual dysfunction.
   - d.   a nonprogressive neuromotor disorder.

2.   Which of the following may cause cerebral palsy?
   - a.   hemorrhage
   - b.   anoxia
   - c.   trauma
   - d.   all of the above

3.   The incidence of cerebral palsy is
   - a.   1.5 children per 2,000 births
   - b.   2 children per 1,500 births
   - c.   1.5 to 2 children per 1000 births
   - d.   1.5 children per 1,500 births

4.   The premature liver secretes a substance called
   - a.   jaundice
   - b.   bilirubin
   - c.   hemoglobin
   - d.   substantia nigra

5.   Which of the following neuromotor disorders is not sen in cerebral palsy?
   - a.   hypotonia
   - b.   spasticity
   - c.   dyskinesia
   - d.   ataxia

6.   Which of the following muscular conditions is related to the individual's emotional state?
   - a.   spasticity
   - b.   tension
   - c.   hypotonicity
   - d.   athetosis

7. A generalized increase in muscle tone when considerable physical effort is exerted is called...
    a. athetosis
    b. chorea
    c. ataxia
    d. overflow
8. The cerebellum is the part of the brain considered essential to...
    a. control of stretch reflex
    b. initiation of movement
    c. coordination of synergistic muscles
    d. inhibition of movement
9. Hyperactivity of reflexes is characteristic of which form of neuromotor dysfunction?
    a. spasticity
    b. dyskinesia
    c. ataxia
    d. hypokinesia
10. What term describes spastic involvement of the legs with little or no involvement of oral or upper extremity musculature?
    a. diplegia
    b. quadriplegia
    c. paraplegia
    d. hemiplegia
11. What is the typical respiratory dysfunction in cerebra palsy?
    a. to much force in exhalation
    b. inhalatory stridor
    c. reduction in the amount of air inhalation and exhalation
    d. low respiratory rate
12. What is the physician's role in management of cerebral palsy?
    a. establishment of initial diagnosis and monitoring health
    b. evaluation of learning potential and adjustment patterns
    c. longitudinal observation of the child's communication behavior
    d. assist with the problems of upper extremity involvement and daily living
13. Which pioneering neurologist recognized subgroups within the diagnosis of cerebral palsy?
    a. Sigmund Freud
    b. W.J. Little
    c. A. Gesell
    d.. K.L. Blackman
14. Which of the following occurs most infrequently in cerebral palsy?
    a. hypertonia
    b. flaccidity
    c. hypotonia
    d. ataxia

15. As many as one third of patients who have spasticity or dyskinesia show signs of...
    a. mixed type
    b. chorea
    c. tremor
    d. ataxia

16. What is a likely developmental course for infantile reflexes in children with cerebral palsy?
    a. They disappear too early.
    b. They are retained and exaggerated.
    c. They move to the lower extremity only.
    d. They become more primitive.

17. What type of paralysis involves the upper and lower extremities of only one side of the body
    a. diplegia
    b. hemiplegia
    c. quadriplegia
    d. paraplegia

18. Monotony of speech is a sign of...
    a. dysprosody.
    b. respiratory dysfunction.
    c. hemiplegia
    d. imprecise consonant articulation.

19. Which Public Law prohibits discrimination against persons with disabilities?
    a. IDEA
    b. EEOC
    c. Affirmative Action
    d. ADA

20. Which type of AAC device is probably best for individuals with limited intellectual abilities?
    a. digitized speech
    b. low-tech system
    c. synthesized speech
    d. row-column scanning

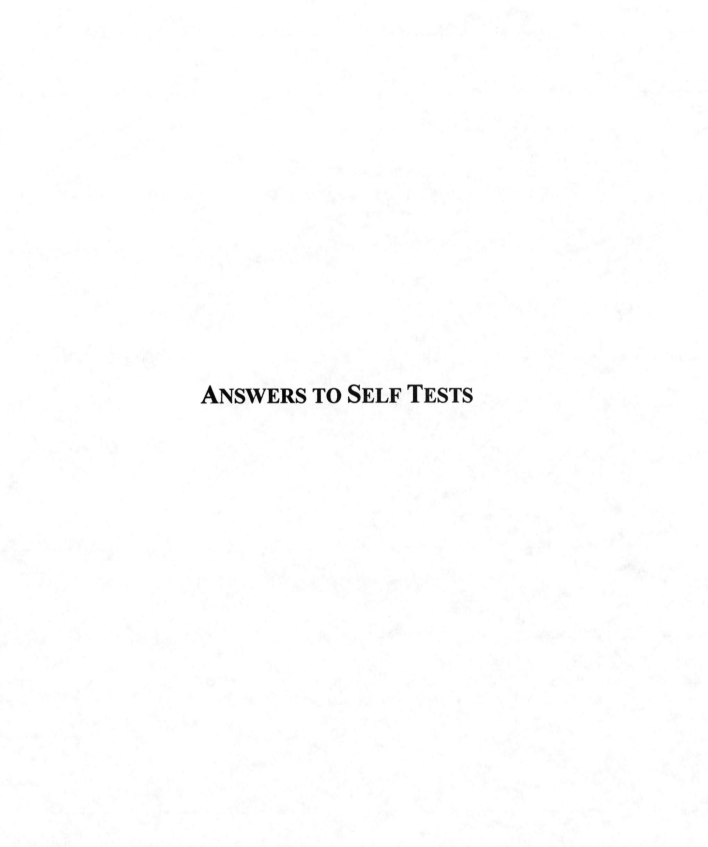

ANSWERS TO SELF TESTS

Answers to Self Test: Chapter One

The Professions of Speech-Language Pathology and Audiology

Fred Spahr and Russ Malone

True/False

1.   The titles, "Speech-Language Pathologist" and "Audiologist " describe the same professionals.
       True
       False o
2.   Most professions describe and enforce their own ethical codes.
       True o
       False
3.   Once professional standards are established, they remain never change.
       True
       False o
4.   Communication disorders have no economic impact in the United States..
       True
       False o
5.   Audiologists are health care professionals who specialize in swallowing disorders.
       True
       False o
6.   Hearing loss can be prevented.
       True o
       False
7.   Audiological assessment can only be performed with adult patients
       True
       False o
8.   A hearing aid can cure a hearing loss.
       True
       False o
9.   A rehabilitation team directs the person with the hearing loss.
       True
       False o
10.   Speech-Language Pathologists provide remedial services to people with voice disorders..
       True o
       False
11.   Dysphagia is a loss or impairment of language following brain damage.
       True
       False o
12.   Speech-Language Pathologists help people whose voices are too hoarse.
       True o
       False

13. Articulation disorders may distract the listener.
    True o
    False
14. A speech or language disorder may signal the onset of a "stroke."
    True o
    False
15. All speech scientists may be employed by private laboratories
    True o
    False
16. Disordered articulation may be associated with a medical condition.
    True o
    False
17. The prevalence of communication disorders is increasing in the United States.
    True o
    False
18. In 1995, over one half of speech-language pathologists worked in schools.
    True o
    False
19. The Master's degree is needed to practice Audiology or Speech-Language Pathology.
    True o
    False
20. Professional Licensure in all 50 of the United States is managed by the American Speech-Language and Hearing Association..
    True
    False o

Multiple Choice

1. Which of the following is *not* characteristic of a profession?
    a.   A profession is a highly paid employment opportunity. o
    b.   A profession delineates its areas of function.
    c.   A profession determines and continues to raise standards of competence of its members.
    d.   A profession develops a distinct body of information.
2. Which organization represents both speech-language pathologists and audiologists?
    a.   The American Speech-Language and Hearing Association. o
    b.   The Acoustic Society of America.
    c.   The American Academy of Audiology.
    d.   The Council of Supervisors in Speech-Language Pathology and Audiology.
3. Speech-Language and Hearing scientists may be employed at...
    a.   Universities
    b.   Private Laboratories.
    c.   Government Agencies.
    d.   All of the above. o
4. Which of the following people are regularly exposed to potentially damaging noise?
    a.   Librarians
    b.   Swimmers
    c.   Home Owners Doing Yard Work o
    d.   Ministers

5. Which of the following is way to prevent hearing loss??
    a. Education.
    b. Wearing Hearing Protection.
    c. Avoiding Ototoxic Drugs.
    d. All of the Above. ○

6. The effects of hearing loss on normal language development will be minimized if...
    a. A child is male.
    b. A child is from a high income family
    c. The hearing loss is identified early. ○
    d. English is the primary language.

7. Audiologists are employed by industry to...
    a. Ensure compliance with OSHA standards
    b. Establishing prevention and early detection programs.
    c. Dispensing hearing aids in the workplace.
    d. All of the Above. ○

8. A conscious effort to simulate a hearing loss when one does not exist is called...
    a. *Malingering* ○
    b. A Conductive Hearing Loss
    c. Sensorineural Hearing Loss.
    d. Audition.

9. A physician who specialized in diseases of the ear is called a/an...
    a. Gastroenterologist
    b. Otologist. ○
    c. Urologist.
    d. Neurologist.

10. Which two speech sounds might cause confusion for speech readers?
    a. /s/ and /h/.
    b. /p/ and /b/. ○
    c. /l/ and /m/.
    d. /f/ and /p/.

11. Which of the following has the most important place on a rehabilitation team along with a Speech-Language Pathologist and an Audiologist?
    a. Medical Doctor
    b. The Person with the Hearing Loss and Her Family. ○
    c. Psychologist
    d. Educational Specialist

12. Difficulty with expression and comprehension of language across all the language channels is...
    a. Dysarthria.
    b. Aphasia. ○
    c. Dysphagia.
    d. Dysgraphia

13. Voice disorders may include
    a. Breathiness
    b. Hoarseness
    c. Low Pitch
    d. All of the above ○

14. The most effective means of preventing Speech and language problems in children is...
   a. Information and Counseling. ○
   b. Therapy.
   c. Diet.
   d. Surgery.
15. Which of the following might need the services of an Audiologist?
   a. crack babies
   b. yard workers
   c. rock musicians
   d. all of the above ○

Answers to Self Test Chapter Two

Development of Communication, Language and Speech

Robert E. Owens, Jr.

<u>True/False</u>

1.   Language is a conventional system of symbols.
      True   o
      False

2.   In most children, communicative development is a phenomenon related to, but separate from speech development.
      True   o
      False

3.   *This Little Piggy* is an example of a joint action routine.
      True   o
      False

4.   Development of the intonation patterns in speech reflect maturation of the paralinguistic aspect of communication.
      True
      False   o

5.   The form or structure of a sentence is governed by syntactic rules.
      True   o
      False

6.   Phonological rules govern the meaning and relationships between meaning units.
      True
      False   o

7.   The smallest unit of grammar is an morpheme.
      True   o
      False

8.   Word knowledge precedes language.
      True   o
      False

9.   Repetition strings of the same consonant-vowel combinations, such as *bababa*, are called reduplications.
      True   o
      False

10. Early words are learned receptively and then produced expressively.
      True   o
      False

11. A *bound* morpheme can function independently in a sentence.
      True
      False   o

12. Pragmatic rules govern speech acts.
   True o
   False
13. Most children have learned 90% of adult syntax by the time they have entered kindergarten.
   True o
   False
14. A child's lexicon is a personal dictionary.
   True o
   False
15. Native speakers of a language learn the permissible rule combinations of that language.
   True o
   False
16. Free morphemes are independent and can be used independently.
   True
   False
17. Most toddlers learn verbs before they learn nouns.
   True
   False o
18. Many experts believe that imitation forms the roots of symbolic function.
   True o
   False
19. The order of consonant acquisition can be predicted by the frequency of their usage or appearance in a child's native language.
   True
   False o
20. Traditional classification of vowels is by place and manner of articulation.
   True
   False o
21. Bilabial consonants are the easiest for a child to articulate.
   True o
   False
22. Phonological rules govern sound distribution and sequencing.
   True o
   False
23. Speech development appears related to increased control over oral muscles.
   True o
   False
24. English consonants which differ only in terms of voicing are called cognates.
   True o
   False

Multiple Choice

1. Communication involves the active processes of :
   a. Syntax, semantics, phonology.
   b. Place, manner, voicing.
   c. Encoding, transmitting, decoding. o
   d. Intonation, stress, rate.

2. Bloom and Lahey (1978) described language as:
    a. A socially shared code. ०
    b. Words, sentences, and paragraphs.
    c. The native tongue of an entire country.
    d. A messaging system.
3. Which aspect of language is concerned with permissible sound combinations?
    a. Pragmatics
    b. Morphology
    d. Phonology ०
    e. Semantics
4. The science of word meaning is called:
    a. Syntax
    b. Semantics ०
    c. Pragmatics
    d. Metalinguistics
5. Linguistic meaning units are called:
    a. Morphemes ०
    b. Phonemes
    c. Acts
    d. Allophones
6. Small changes in speech sounds that are not sufficient to change word meaning are called:
    a. Phonemic
    b. Sound families
    c. Metalinguistic
    d. Allophonic ०
7. The earliest communication between care-giver and child probably involves:
    a. Guttural oral sounds
    b. Head movements and gaze patterns ०
    c. A shared system of symbols, signs, or actions
    d. Turn taking
8. The earliest use of verbal intentions normally appears by the:
    a. First month of life.
    b. Sixth month of life.
    c. First year of life.
    d. Second year of life. ०
9. Paralinguistic, nonlinguistic and metalinguistic communication makes its greatest developmental strides during which stage of life?
    a. The sixth month.
    b. The preschool period.
    c. The metaphonemic stage.
    d. The school-age. ०
10. A language user's underlying knowledge about a linguistic rule system may be called:
    a. Linguistic competence. ०
    b. Morphophonemic transference
    c. Allophonic variation.
    d. Metalinguistic relativism
11. Language use may described as :
    a. Content
    b. Function
    c. Pragmatics ०
    d. Form

12. Syntactic rules govern:
    a. The order of sequential linguistic units. ○
    b. The meaning of linguistic units
    c. The list of permissible speech sounds.
    d. Long-distance telephone rates for a region.
13. Body posture, facial expression and physical proximity are clues in which aspects of communication?
    a. Nonlinguistic ○
    b. Paralinguistic
    c. Metalinguistic
    d. Phonological
14. What process enables a speaker to use language knowledge to produce more language?:
    a. Joint attention
    b. Turn taking
    c. Joint reference
    d. Bootstrapping ○
15. What do linguists call the phonological changes that occur when speakers join certain morphemes?
    a. Semantic
    b. Bootstrapping
    c. Morphophonemic ○
    d. Metalinguistic
16. Adult-like use of stress of emphasis in speech is mastered by which age?
    a. Infant
    b. Toddler
    c. School-age ○
    d. Adult
17. Words that share identical semantic features are called...
    a. Homonyms
    b. Antonyms
    c. Synonyms ○
    d. Pseudonyms
18. Which speech sounds require a closed or constricted vocal tract passage?
    a. Vowels
    b. Diphthongs
    c. Monophthongs
    d. Consonants ○
19. Psycholinguists attempt to explain...
    a. Syntactic rules.
    b. The relationship between language form and cognitive processing. ○
    c. Speech articulation development.
    d. Morphological principles.
20. Which parts of speech predominate the vocabularies of most toddlers?
    a. Nouns ○
    b. Verbs
    c. Prepositions
    d. Adverbs
21. Subphoneme units of speech sound analysis are called:
    a. Distinctive features ○
    b. Lip rounding, place, and tenseness
    c. Manner, place, and voicing
    d. Free variation

22. Which of the following is an aspect of the traditional consonant phoneme classification system?
    a. Allophonic variation
    b. Strident deletion
    c. Manner of articulation o
    d. Tense/lax
23. When a child's word meaning features contain more examples than the adult meaning, they are called:
    a. Underextensions
    b. Overextensions o
    c. Metaextensions
    d. Betaextensions
24. A grammatic form that contains both a noun and a verb is called a...
    a. Predicate
    b. Subject
    c. Modifier
    d. Clause o
25. Saying "wawa " for "water" is an example of which phonological processes?
    a. Reduplication o
    b. Assimilation
    c. Deletion of unstressed syllables
    d. Reduction of consonant clusters
26. The developmental stage in which a child appears to experiment with sounds through long periods of vocalizing strings of meaningless sounds is called...
    a. The experimenting stage
    b. Phonotactics
    c. Substitution
    d. Babbling o

True/False

1. There is a wide a span of human anatomical attributes called "normal.".
    > True o
    > False

2. The larynx is built to withstand prolonged yelling.
    > True
    > False o

3. We inhale by creating negative air pressure in the lungs:
    > True o
    > False

4. Increased tension of in the vocal folds is usually accompanied by an increase in pitch.
    > True o
    > False

5. The diaphragm is a muscle of exhalation.
    > True
    > False o

6. The upper portion of the trunk is called the *abdomen*.
    > True
    > False o

7. The vocal tract consists of the pharynx, oral cavity and nasal cavity.
    > True o
    > False

8. Consonants are produced with a relatively open vocal tract.
    > True
    > False o

9. The larynx excites the air in the upper respiratory tract.
    > True o
    > False

10. Whispered vowels are always voiced.
    > True
    > False o

11. The respiratory tract begins at the mouth and nose and ends deep in the lungs.
    > True o
    > False

12. When we are not talking, we breathe quietly about twelve times each minute.
    True o
    False
13. The thorax contains the lungs.
    True o
    False
14. Most consonants require vibration of the vocal folds.
    True o
    False
15. The biomechanics of speech breathing are similar to those for vegetative breathing.
    True
    False o
16. Muscular force for exhalation is never required during speech.
    True
    False o
17. The diaphragm is a muscle of exhalation.
    True
    False o
18. We use our tidal respiratory volume during quiet breathing.
    True o
    False
19. The average vital capacity in adults ranges from 1000 to 1500 cc.
    True o
    False
20. The largest of the laryngeal cartilages is the thyroid cartilage.
    True o
    False
21. The permanent teeth are also known as the deciduous teeth.
    True
    False o
22. The cricothyroid muscle opposes the thyroarytenoid muscle.
    True o
    False
23. When the posterior cricoarytenoid muscles contract, the glottis becomes larger.
    True o
    False
24. The orbicularis oris muscle purses the lips.
    True o
    False
25. When the genioglossus muscle contracts, the tongue moves forward.
    True o
    False
26. The lower jaw is called the maxilla.
    True
    False o
27. The pharynx is a dynamic articulator.
    True
    False o
28. The velum is lowered for production of /m/.
    True o
    False

29. A vowel produced with the tongue held high and forward will probably be recognized as /i/.
        True ○
        False
30. Voiced speech sounds are shaped by alterations in the configuration of the vocal tract.
        True ○
        False
31. The cranial nerves are located along the spinal cord.
        True
        False ○
32. The peripheral nervous system is contained in the skull and spinal column.
        True
        False ○
33. The temporal lobe is part of the forebrain.
        True ○
        False
34. Broca discovered that 90% of people who had damage to Broca's area on the left side also had aphasia.
        True ○
        False
35. We are born with an estimated 100 billion neurons.
        True ○
        False

Multiple Choice

1. The amount of air remaining in the lungs after a maximum exhalation is called:
        a. vital capacity
        b. functional reserve volume
        c. residual volume ○
        d. complemental air.
2. Which of the following is included among the human vocal organs?
        a. eyes
        b. ears
        c. larynx ○
        d. heart
3. A fairly regular series of air pulses is produced by the larynx during:
        a. phonation ○
        b. pronation
        c. phonetics
        d. phonics
4. An important role of hearing in normal speech is one of:
        a. reaction to danger
        b. maintenance of balance
        c. triggering the stapedial reflex
        d. providing feedback ○
5. During the speech act, the muscles of muscles of inhalation perform which function?
        a. partially defeat excessive relaxation pressure ○
        b. produce micro-movements for phonation
        c. draw air into the lungs
        d. increase airflow rate during utterance of stressed syllables

6. Neurogenic respiratory disorders may result in:
   a. lack of control of inhalation
   b. inability to switch from vegetative to speech breathing
   c. inappropriate active exhalation
   d. all of the above ○

7. The muscle thought to be primarily responsible for shortening and opposing tension on the vocal folds is the:
   a. posterior cricoarytenoid
   b. lateral cricoarytenoid
   c. cricothyroid
   d. thyroarytenoid ○

8. The laryngeal cartilage shaped like a ring is the:
   a. cricoid ○
   b. epiglottis
   c. arytenoid
   d. thyroid

9. The vocal ligaments attach to which part of each arytenoid cartilage?
   a. muscular process
   b. vocal process ○
   c. cricothyroid process
   d. apex

10. The function of the posterior cricoarytenoid muscles is to:
    a. adduct the vocal ligaments
    b. abduct the vocal ligaments ○
    c. increase tension on the vocal ligaments
    d. decrease tension in the vocal ligaments

11. A muscle important in increasing tension of the vocal folds is the:
    a. posterior cricoarytenoid
    b. lateral cricoarytenoid
    c. thyroarytenoid
    d. cricothyroid ○

12. Adult female vocal folds vibrate at about:
    a. 65 times per second
    b. 10,000 times per second
    c. 120-145 times per second
    d. 200-260 times per second ○

13. The *Rima Glottidis* is:
    a. the pharynx
    b. the space between the teeth and the cheeks
    d. the space between the true margins of the vocal folds ○
    e. the oral cavity

14. Which of the following may affect the sound of the voice?:
    a. medial compression, longitudinal tension and subglottic pressure ○
    b. smoking alcohol and polluted air
    c. mass changes caused by inflammation of the vocal folds
    d. all of the above ○

15. The functional cells of the nervous system are called :
    a. glial cells
    b. neurons ○
    c. oligodendroglia
    d. end brushes

394

16. Raised areas on the surface of the cerebrum are called:
    a. nuclei
    b. gyri o
    c. sulci
    d. ventricles
17. Speech is what kind of respiratory function??
    a. digestive
    b. circulatory
    c. respiratory o
    d. biosocial
18. In which part of the brain are the cranial nerve nuclei located?
    a. forebrain and basal ganglia
    b. midbrain and hindbrain o
    c. cerebellum
    d. corpus callosum
19. The vocal tract behave acoustically like a:
    a. a tube, closed at one end and open at the other o
    b. a box with no top
    c. a pair of strings, anchored at both ends
    d. a reed
20. The resonances of the vocal tract are called:
    a. fundamentals
    b. formants o
    c. overtones
    d. volume
21. On which vertebra does the skull rest?:
    a. Vertebra Prominens
    b. Atlas o
    c. Axis
    d. T-12
22. Deciduous teeth are commonly called:
    a. permanent teeth
    b. "baby teeth" o
    c. front teeth
    d. molars
23. The roof of the oral cavity is formed by parts of the .
    a. mandible
    b. maxilla o
    c. velum
    d. thyroid
24. The nasal and pharyngeal cavities are coupled through action of the:
    a. maxilla
    b. epiglottis
    c. velum o
    d. all of the above
25. The opening between the true margins of the vocal folds is called the:
    a. epiglottis
    b. glottis o
    c. pharynx
    d. none of the above

26. Approximation of the vocal folds is called:
    a. medial compression ○
    b. longitudinal tension
    c. phonation
    d. subglottal air pressure

27. The three divisions of the pharynx are:
    a. vestibule, ventricle and subglottic area
    b. nasopharynx, oropharynx and laryngopharynx ○
    c. labiopharynx, linguopharynx and glottidopharynx
    d. frontal, parietal and occipital

28. Cognate pairs differ in terms of which feature?
    a. manner of articulation
    b. tongue placement
    c. presence or absence of phonation ○
    d. tongue height

29. The muscle that protrudes the tongue is called:
    a. palatoglossus
    b. hyoglossus
    c. genioglossus ○
    d. linguoglossus

30. The muscles that move the mandible can be grouped functionally into:
    a. elevators
    b. depressors
    c. a protractor
    d. all of the above ○

31. The articulators change the shape (and acoustic characteristics) of the vocal tract in which of the following dimensions?
    a. overall length
    b. location of constriction
    c. degree of constriction
    d. all of the above ○

32. The vowel /u/ may be described as:
    a. close front
    b. close back ○
    c. open front
    d. open back

33. A blend of two separate vowels may be called a:
    a. close front vowel
    b. monophthong
    c. diphthong ○
    d. triphthong

34. The places of consonant articulation include:
    a. mandibular
    b. labiodental ○
    c. cranial
    d. orbicular

35. Sounds generated with rapid articulatory movement, and without prominent noise or turbulence are called:
    a. diphthongs
    b. affricates
    c. homophones
    d. glides ○

True/False

1. Cultural groups may vary in several aspects of language use.
    True o
    False

2. Dialects of a language include deep structure as well as surface structure.
    True o
    False

3. The terms *regional dialects* and *accent* have the same meaning.
    True
    False o

4. Dialects and accents are language disorders.
    True
    False o

5. If a dialect results in ridicule of the speaker, it is a communication disorder.
    True o
    False

6. Culture is learned.
    True o
    False

7. Standardized language proficiency tests are relatively valid if the cultural background of the person being tested is represented in the test's standardization sample.
    True o
    False

8. Culture may be represented by standards for health and hygiene.
    True o
    False

9. Members of the same race may have different cultures.
    True o
    False

10. Dialects of social groups are easily changed by outside forces.
    True
    False o

11. Ethnic influences on language are basically biological in nature.
    True
    False o

12. Individuals may speak several dialects.
> True o
> False

13. Membership in a cultural group is a good predictor of language form.
> True
> False o

14. Inhabitants of a geographic region belong to the same speech community.
> True
> False o

15. Child rearing styles may affect meal length of utterance in children.
> True o
> False

16. The Creolist Theory is currently accepted by all sociolinguists.
> True
> False o

17. Sociolinguists recognize three regional dialects in the continental United States.
> True
> False o

18. Some phonological characteristics of Southern White Nonstandard English are also characteristic of African American English .
> True o
> False

19. Gender is not related to language use.
> True
> False o

20. Code-switching enables a speaker to use more than one language or dialect.
> True o
> False

21. Situation or context may have an effect on language use.
> True o
> False

22. Standard English is "White" English.
> True
> False o

23. Bilingual speakers may code switch as a situation demands.
> True o
> False

24. African American phonology may substitute voiceless labiodental fricatives where voiceless interdental fricatives occur in the standard dialect.
> True o
> False

25. Culture has no discernable effect on stuttering characteristics
> True
> False o

26. According to ASHA policy, accent reduction is outside the scope of practice of speech-language pathologists.
> True
> False o

Multiple Choice

1. The Creole theory suggests that African American English derived from which of the following languages?
   a. Dutch
   b. French
   c. English
   d. all of the above and more ○

2. Which of the following is not a component of *accent*:
   a. semantics ○
   b. phonology
   c. suprasegmental characteristics
   d. vocal characteristics

3. Individuals who speak two languages are said to be:
   a. biglossal.
   b. bicyclical.
   c. bidialectical.
   d. bilingual. ○

4. Variations within a language that include deep structure and linguistic codes are termed:
   a. dialects ○
   b. accents
   c. vernaculars
   d. narratives

5. Which of the following influences language and communication?
   a. ethnicity
   b. social class
   c. gender
   d. all of the above ○

6. Which of the following is a regional dialect?
   a. Creole
   b. African American
   c. Asian American
   d. Southern American ○

7. Which of the following speech differences have investigators associated with gender?
   a. mean length of utterance
   b. type-token ratio
   c. joking ○
   d. lying

8. According to the author, which of the following distinguishes Standard (American) English from its dialectical variants?
   a. deep structure
   b. use of pronouns
   c. linguistic and structural characteristics
   d. vocal patterns, phrase and word and phrase emphases ○

9. Research has shown that simultaneous acquisition of two languages may occur without negative interaction prior to what age?:
   a. 21 years
   b. 3 years ○
   c. 12 years
   d. 30 years

10. African American English s the linguistic code used by:
   a. Africans
   b. all African Americans
   c. Southern Americans
   d. working-class African Americans ○

11. The majority of African American utterances conform to the rules of
   a. Creole English
   b. Appalachian English
   c. Southern American English
   d. General American English

12. Who is among a small group of scholars who account for the full range of language use by African American people in the United States?
   a. K. Payne
   b. O. Taylor ○
   c. W. Secord
   d. E. Wiig

13. The largest group of in the United States today with native language influence on English consists of people from which background?
   a. French
   b. Hebrew
   c. Scottish
   d. Spanish ○

14. Oral-based cultures value:
   a. literature
   b. poetry ○
   c. speech
   d. all of the above

15. Which of the following type of stories is used by working-class children?
   a. topic associated ○
   b. standardized
   c. fairy tales
   d. historical

16. Most of the standardized tests used by speech-language pathologists are based on which variant of American English?
   a. Northern Midland
   b. New York
   c. Southwestern
   d. African American

17. Mismatch between the rules of communication interaction between the test maker and the test taker may be termed:
   a. social/situational bias
   b. phonological bias
   c. pragmatic bias
   d. format bias ○

18. Which of the following is a good solution to standardized test bias?
   a. Never use standardize tests in an evaluation.
   b. Develop criterion-references tests. ○
   c. Publish African American versions of all standardized tests.
   d. Limit evaluation sessions to thirty minutes.

19. "I might could'a done it," is an example of a:
   a. relative clause
   b. intensifying adverb
   c. consonant cluster reduction
   d. double modal ○

20. Age, education, and situation typically influence:
   a. code-switching efficacy are ○
   b. gender, race, and socioeconomic status
   c. region, intelligence, and personality
   d. none of the above.

21. The "Ann Arbor Decision" (1977) outlawed which of the following?
   a. use of dialect in public schools
   b. failure to place culturally different children in speech therapy
   c. inappropriate placement in treatment based on language differences ○
   d. use of standardized tests

22. Which of the following is a characteristic of men's language?
   a. precise articulation
   b. apologizing
   c. profanity in formal mixed company ○
   d. avoiding confrontation

True/False

1. About 75% of school children have speech, language or hearing disorders.
   - True
   - False o

2. The semantic revolution was rooted in the cognitive theories of Piaget.
   - True o
   - False

3. Standardized language tests are useful for making decisions about eligibility.
   - True o
   - False

4. The pragmatic approach to language function emphasizes the social utility of language.
   - True o
   - False

5. Language development is independent of contextual considerations.
   - True
   - False o

6. The psychological well-being of the caregiver has little or no influence on a child's successful language acquisition.
   - True
   - False o

7. A secondary language disorder is presumed to be caused by biological factors.
   - True o
   - False

8. Cerebral palsy is an example of a biological risk factor for language disorders.
   - True o
   - False

9. Child maltreatment can include failure of caregivers to produce a stimulating environment.
   - True o
   - False

10. The severity of a communication disorder cannot be easily predicted from known risk factors.
    - True o
    - False

11. Discourse is the ability to connect one sentence to another.
    - True o
    - False

12. The effects of brain injury on an infant brain may be reliably inferred from observations of similar injuries on adult brains.
    - True
    - False o

13. A child with a measured IQ in the range of 50-70 is considered mentally disabled.
    True o
    False

14. Mental disability is diagnosed according to intellect and adaptation skills.
    True o
    False

15. Echolalia may be a language learning strategy for children with pervasive developmental disorders.
    True o
    False

16. Both cerebral hemispheres have the capacity to learn language.
    True o
    False

17. Early intervention programs for children with language delays should begin before age four.
    True o
    False

18. Federal law provides financial incentives for developing language stimulation programs for infants and toddlers.
    True o
    False

19. Hart and Risley (1995) found no difference in home stimulation associated with socioeconomic status.
    True
    False o

20. Federal regulations require establishment of an Individualized Family Service Plan
    True o
    False

21. Assessment refers to the process used to determine a child's eligibility for treatment services.
    True
    False o

22. Criterion-referenced measures measure a child's level of performance in a specific domain.
    True o
    False

23. Early assessment tools are limited in scope.
    True o
    False

24. Inclusive treatment programs limit opportunities for typical peer interaction.
    True
    False o

25. Whole language approaches integrate all language modalities.
    True o
    False

26. The ultimate goal of language intervention is to make the child a more effective communicator and learner.
    True o
    False

27. Inclusive education is mandated by public law.
    True o
    False

28. Children benefit from predictability and structure.
    True o
    False

29. Drawing is an early form of writing.
    True o
    False

30. Current research supports milieu intervention as the best language teaching approach.

 True
 False o

Multiple Choice:

1. The perspective of language development that emphasizes role of language in ordering a child's environment is the
   a. the grammatical approach.
   b. the transactional approach.
   c. the constructivist approach. o
   d. the interpretive approach.

2. A primary language impairment may be caused by:
   a. visual impairment.
   b. orofacial paralysis.
   c. mental retardation.
   d. none of the above. o

3. The most widely used diagnostic system in the medical profession is:
   a. Diagnostic and Statistical manual of Mental Disorders: IV. o
   b. Merck's Manual.
   c. Burros Mental Measurements Yearbook.
   d. Manual of Medical Professions.

4. The most notable language characteristics of children with SLI include...
   a. echolalia.
   b. adolescent onset.
   c. semantic and grammatical deficits. o
   d. intellectual and adaptive delays.

5. One of the best determinants of a child's outcome is...
   a. age of onset.
   b. the combined number of risk factors. o
   c. maternal health.
   d. socioeconomic status of the family.

6. For children under age three, which is better used for assessment of mental disabilities?
   a. measure of developmental functioning o
   b. a standardized intelligence test
   c. parent questionnaire
   d. all of the above

7. Intelligence quotients below 20 are classified as:
   a. mildly retarded
   b. moderately retarded
   c. severely retarded
   d. profoundly retarded o

8. In children with PDD, what may pronoun reversal signify?
   a. rejection of the caregiver
   b. mental retardation
   c. use of language learning strategy o
   d. sensory deficits.

7. Swelling and edema following brain injury can lead to:
   a. generalized symptoms ∘
   b. focal deficits
   c. specific language impairment
   d. Broca's aphasia.

8. Special educational programs in the schools are documented which form?
   a. Health Care Finance Administration form #700.
   b. Individual Family Service Plan.
   c. Individual Educational Program. ∘
   d. clinical progress notes.

9. The process of determining a child's eligibility for services includes:
   a. standardized test scores ∘
   b. assessment protocols
   c. curriculum planning
   d. plan of treatment

10. Ongoing procedures used to identify the child's strengths and needs are part of which process?
    a. assessment ∘
    b. evaluation
    c. I.Q. testing
    d. achievement testing

11. An intelligence quotient is usually inferred from which type of measurement?
    a. performance assessment
    b. criterion referenced testing
    c. informal assessment
    d. norm referenced testing ∘

12. Validity of parental reports are greatly enhanced under which circumstances?
    a. The parents are allowed to report as a team.
    b. Parents have high socioeconomic status.
    c. Parents are given an inventory and focus on current skills. ∘
    d. Parents are interviewed separately.

13. The normal age for emerging discourse is:
    a. 6 months
    b. 12 months ∘
    c. 18 months
    d. 24 months

14. What is the role of the teacher in curricular planning?
    a. establish eligibility for speech therapy
    b. establish treatment goals and objectives
    c. prepare the learning environment and plan experiences ∘
    d. supervise the speech-language pathologist

15. Using themes to enhance concept development is called what?
    a. theme building ∘
    b. whole language approach
    c. direct teaching
    d. pull-out therapy

16. What is probably the most important time to begin inclusion?
    a. infancy
    b. early childhood
    c. adolescence
    d. There is never a good time to begin inclusion.

17. Which modality is emphasized in a whole language approach?
    a. spoken language
    b. written language
    c. gestural language
    d. all of the above ○

18. In language stimulation, what does "JAR" mean?
    a. joined activity regulation
    b. joint action routine ○
    c. Treatment objectives are written down and placed in a small glass container.
    d. Treatment results come as a surprise to the clinician and the child.

19. Typical and atypical children learn in the same classroom in which model?
    a. segregative model
    b. integrative model
    c. joint action routine
    d inclusive model ○

20. Through which teaching method does the teacher systematically present stimuli, elicit an expected response and provide consistent consequences?
    a. direct teaching ○
    b. inclusion
    c. incidental teaching
    d. milieu intervention

21. What does scaffolding provide for a child learning language?
    a. grammar
    b. contextual support ○
    c. incidental teaching
    d. success

22. Literacy begins at which developmental stage?
    a. infancy ○
    b. early childhood
    c. elementary school age
    d. adolescence

23. Which teaching technique has been established as superior?
    a. direct teaching
    b. indirect teaching
    c. milieu intervention
    d. none of the above ○

24. Which public law mandates family centered practice?
    a. 94-142
    b. 99-457
    c. IDEA
    d. 101-457

25. Which of the following are part of the process of grieving?
    a. denial
    b. anxiety
    c. guilt
    d. all of the above. ○

True/False

1. A child cannot learn to read or write fluently if the native language has not been learned adequately.
   - True o
   - False

2. By legal definition, children with learning disabilities have problems in all academic areas.
   - True
   - False o

3. There is a high incidence of brain injury among children with LLD.
   - True o
   - False

4. The most common learning disability syndrome is termed *language disorder syndrome* (language-learning disabilities).
   - True o
   - False

5. If intervention has not begun by third grade, it is to late to help the LLD child.
   - True
   - False o

6. Language learning disabilities may appear in 5% of all children diagnosed as learning disabled.
   - True
   - False o

7. Children and adolescents with *visuospatial perceptual deficit syndrome* have difficulty with visually oriented tasks.
   - True o
   - False

8. Children with ADD may not be hyperactive.
   - True o
   - False

9. Nondominant hemisphere dysfunction may affect reasoning, social perception and inner language
   - True o
   - False

10. Learning disabilities have no genetic basis.
    - True
    - False o

11. The primary language processing area in the left cerebral hemisphere is known as Wernicke's area.
    - True o
    - False

12. Once a child grows into adolescence, it is too late for effective language therapy.
    - True
    - False o

13. Children with language-learning disabilities often have difficulty recognizing verbal patterns in communication.

        True ○
        False

14. Classroom scripts develop in an ongoing process.

        True ○
        False

15. Children with language disabilities generally have difficulty with text comprehension.

        True ○
        False

16. Children with LLD may earn lower grades because they lack the ability to control narrative structure.

        True ○
        False

17. It would not be unusual for a student with LLD to score normally on a picture vocabulary test.

        True ○
        False

18. Traumatic brain injury may disrupt use of all acquired linguistic skills.

        True ○
        False

19. Most immigrants and persons from culturally diverse backgrounds display characteristics of language-learning disabilities.

        True
        False ○

20. Portfolio assessment is a form of performance assessment.

        True ○
        False

21. Strategy-based intervention uses passive techniques.

        True ○
        False

22. Students with LLD use common scripts for daily life functions, but must be supported to recognize classroom scripts.

        True
        False ○

23. Whole-language approaches emphasize choosing one language modality appropriate to a communicative situation.

        True
        False ○

24. Language intervention should be the only treatment required for language learning deficits.

        True
        False ○

25. The inclusion movement emphasizes that teachers must help students develop self-image.

        True ○
        False

Multiple Choice

1. Language learning disabilities may affect performance in which of the following areas?

    a. listening
    b. speaking
    c. writing
    d. all of the above ○

2. The least common deficit syndrome among children and adolescents with specific learning disability is:
    a. visuospatial perceptual deficit o
    b. articulatory and graphomotor dyscoordination syndrome
    c. sensory-motor deficit
    d. language learning disabilities
3. Which area of the brain is primarily implicated in attention deficit disorder?
    a. frontal lobe o
    b. parietal lobe
    c. occipital lobe
    d. temporal lobe
4. Which of the following genetic disorders is associated with learning disabilities?
    a. Turner syndrome o
    b. Marfan's syndrome
    c. Hunter's syndrome
    d. Down syndrome
5. Electrical stimulation of which part of the brain produced disruptions in speech sound discrimination in Ojemann and Mateer's (1979) study?
    a. corpus striatum
    b. left temporal lobe o
    c. right temporal lobe
    d. thalamus
6. Nonverbal learning disabilities are characterized by:
    a. deficient math and reasoning skills
    b. poor visuospatial, organizational, and social perception skills
    c. inadequate social skills
    d. all of the above o
7. When LLD is precipitated by a traumatic brain injury, the disability is said to be:
    a. syndromic
    b. biological
    c. transient
    d. acquired o
8. Which of the following skills is required to use language as a joke?
    a. metalinguistic o
    b. paralinguistic
    c. visual closure
    d. figure-ground discrimination
9. At what age should a child appropriately interpret figurative word use?
    a. two years
    b. five years
    c. thirteen years o
    d. eighteen years
10. Which of the following is among the prerequisites for communication strategy use?
    a. ability to substitute words
    b. ability to switch codes
    c. ability to inhibit responses and reflect o
    d. ability to circumlocute
11. Children with language-learning disabilities often progress to the linguistic transition stages typical for which ages?
    a. three to five years
    b. seven to ten years o
    c. ten to fifteen years
    d. fifteen to twenty years

411

12. The underlying plan of a conversation is called a...
    a. speech
    b. script o
    c. poem
    d. billet doux

13. Stubbs (1993) found which of the following among the cohesive mechanisms for discourse and narrative?
    a. use of synonyms
    b. verbal math skills
    c. ability to follow lexical repetition patterns o
    d. ability to associate a word with a picture

14. Which of the following is the best single indicator of reading achievement?
    a. word knowledge o
    b. sequential memory
    c. pragmatic skills
    d. nonverbal communication

15. What type of word task might we expect to present difficulty to a child with LLD?
    a. matching spoken words to pictures
    b. remembering series of spoken words
    c. saying the antonyms of spoken words o
    d. rhyming spoken words

16. Which of the following semantic cues is/are required for a student to learn the meaning of a new word from text?
    a. its class membership o
    b. its spelling
    c. articulatory posture of its initial sound
    d. all of the above

17. In addition to language therapy, the child with LLD is most likely to need what other type of treatment?
    a. physical therapy
    b. occupational therapy
    c. nursing
    d. counseling o

18. A mature language user responds to perceived needs of listeners through which process?
    a. direction
    b. metalinguistic ability o
    c. paraphrasing
    d. manners

19. The most common effects of closed head injury result from damage to which nervous system structure?
    a. Wernicke's area
    b. Broca's area
    c. basal ganglia
    d. A single focal site usually cannot be identified o

20. Which of the following is a useful communication strategy for students with LLD?
    a. use pictures for redundancy
    b. speak very slowly
    c. use multiple words with the same meaning
    d. reduce complex pragmatic rules to simple, automated ones o

21. The counseling approach in which the counselor shares knowledge to increase the client's understanding is called what?
    a. direct approach o
    b. indirect approach
    c. self-oriented approach
    d. treatment oriented approach

22. Wernicke's area is located in the:
    a. subcortical region
    b. cerebral cortex o
    c. spinal cord
    d. lateral geniculate nucleus
23. Which of the following is an outcome of norm-referenced testing?
    a. Determination of language disability presence
    b. Identify strengths and weaknesses
    c. Determine eligibility for placement
    d. all of the above o
24. Criterion referenced testing can be used to...
    a. determine placement eligibility
    b. compare the subject's performance to a large sample of other children
    c. verify results of norm-referenced testing o
    d. determine the presence of a language disability

Answers to Self Test Chapter Seven

Phonological Disorders

Richard G. Schwartz

True/False

1. Articulation is not a part of phonology.
   - True
   - False o
2. For the best assessment of a child's phonological skills, a speech-language pathologist should look at syllable formation in a variety of contexts
   - True o
   - False
3. A disorder of the motor production system is likely to produce a phonetic disorder
   - True o
   - False
4. For many children, phonological disorders are accompanied by syntactic deficits.
   - True o
   - False
5. Intelligibility refers to how well a child's speech is understood.
   - True o
   - False
6. Phonological disabilities in children with hearing disorders varies with the type and severity of the loss.
   - True o
   - False
7. There is no relationship between intelligence and intelligibility.
   - True
   - False o
8. A phonological disorder is a sure sign of other developmental disorders.
   - True
   - False o
9. Research suggests that children produce nouns more accurately than they produce verbs.
   - True o
   - False
10. Reading seems to be dependent on metaphonological abilities.
    - True o
    - False
11. Signs of general sensory deficits are of no significance in assessment of phonology.
    - True
    - False o
12. Commercially available articulation tests are advantageous in cases where the child's speech is very unintelligible.
    - True
    - False o
13. Phonology describes the contrastive elements in written language.
    - True
    - False o

14. Some children have different sound-contrast systems than adults.

           True o

           False

15. Phonological development stabilized at age five.

           True

           False o

16. A child who "fails" a screening is referred for evaluation.

           True o

           False

17. Most standardized tests allow for cultural variations in children's responses.

           True

           False o

18. Phonological disorders are sure signs of perceptual disorders.

           True

           False o

19. Any child being evaluated for a phonological disorder should receive a complete audiological evaluation.

           True

           False o

20. The maintenance phase of articulation treatment addresses production in conversational speech.

           True o

           False

21. Early forms of phonological treatment focused on distinctive feature training.

           True o

           False

22. The "cycle" approach sets no performance criteria before progression to the next goal.

           True

           False o

23. Therapy frequency may be dictated by the clinician's schedule.

           True o

           False

24. The speech-language pathologist may be considered a natural interactor under most circumstances.

           True

           False o

25. Effective treatment activities must provide the child opportunities to hear correct responses.

           True o

           False

Multiple Choice

1. Which of the following describes *phonology*?
   a. the structure of conversation
   b. the meaning of words and larger units
   c. the structure of words in terms of consonants, vowels, and syllables o
   d. the structure of complex words and inflections

2. Children who have phonological disorders have:
   a. hearing impairments
   b. structural anomalies
   c. motor disorders
   d. linguistic deficits o

3. Phonological disorders are characterized by :
   a. widespread patterns of errors
   b. limitations on syllable structure
   c. limitations in the range of sounds produced
   d. all of the above ○

4. Rapid utterance of a series of syllables is called...
   a. diadochokinesis ○
   b. imitative movement
   c. blathering
   d. balanced movement

5. Clinicians approach "tongue thrust" as a...
   a. phonological disorder
   b. phonetic disorder
   c. swallowing disorder ○
   d. syntactical disorder

6. What is the assumed underlying disability in *developmental apraxia of speech*?
   a. paralysis
   b. linguistic disturbance
   c. auditory perceptual disorder
   d. sequencing motor movements ○

7. What is the relationship between otitis media and phonological disorders?
   a. it is the number one cause of phonological disorder
   b. it has no effect on speech development
   c. the relationship is not clear ○
   d. none of the above

8. In phonological assessment when does diagnosis occur?
   a. during the screening process
   b. after identification ○
   c. after a period of treatment
   d. six months after screening

9. Which of the following is an advantage of commercially available articulation tests?
   a. They provide analysis of phonological systems.
   b. They provide a natural context for evaluation
   c. They provide a way to compare unintelligible speech to the adult target. ○
   d. They have no advantages.

10. The *Kahn-Lewis Phonological Analysis* is intended to be used with which commercial articulation test?
   a. all articulation tests
   b. *Fisher-Logemann Test of Articulation Competence*
   c. *Arizona Articulation Proficiency Scale*
   d. *Goldman-Fristoe Test of Articulation* ○

11. Independent phonological analysis examines a child's...
   a. phonetic inventory ○
   b. phonological processes
   c. approximations of the adult target
   d. distinctive feature analysis

12. Which of the following is inferred through phonological sample analysis?
   a. the child's knowledge of phonology
   b. the child's perceptual abilities
   c. the child's phonetic production abilities
   d. all of the above ○

13.   What is the anterior one-third of the palate called?
         a.   hard palate
         b.   soft palate o
         c.   buccal cavity
         d.   fistulae

14.   What does stimulability for syllables in an imitative context reflect?
         a.   phonetic level perception o
         b.   phonological knowledge
         c.   phonological representation
         d.   phonological organization

15.   What purpose may be served by intelligibility assessment?
         a.   establishment of a measure of functional effects o
         b.   provides a diversion for the child
         c.   may predict the outcome of treatment
         d.   aids in intelligence assessment

16.   Which of the following is the goal of *generalization* in therapy?
         a.   ensure motoric competence
         b.   ensure perceptual ability
         c.   establishment of the phonological act
         d.   ensure changes are systemic phonologically o

17.   A relational sample analysis is an examination of...
         a.   the relationships between a child's productions in different contexts.
         b.   the relationship between the child's production and characteristics of the adult target. o
         c.   the relationship between the adult target and the treatment objective.
         d.   the relationship between the child and the clinician.

18.   What are the focuses of "articulation" approaches to treatment?
         a.   cognitive structure
         b.   phonological abilities
         c.   motor production o
         d.   phonological acquisition

19.   When should a child be dismissed from therapy?
         a.   when speech is 100% intelligible.
         b.   when all goals have been reached at the established criterion level o
         c.   after six months
         d.   when the child reaches age twelve

20.   Which of the following is one of Fey's (1986) dimensions of naturalness?
         a.   treatment materials
         b.   vocal characteristics
         c.   physical context o
         d.   standardization sample

True/False

1. The vocal folds are adducted during quiet respiration.
   - True
   - False o

2. Stutterng is a voice disorder.
   - True
   - False o

3. Vowel contrasts are created by resonance variations.
   - True o
   - False

4. Without a functinal larynx, speech is impossible.
   - True
   - False o

5. All males have roughly the same optimum vocal pitch..
   - True
   - False o

6. Changes in vocal fold mass can affect the sond of the voice.
   - True o
   - False

7. A change in amplitude produces a change in pitch.
   - True
   - False o

8. Most phonemes require a phonatory source.
   - True o
   - False

9. Aphonia is the complete loss of voice.
   - True o
   - False

10. Bilateral vocal fold paralysis is a threat to the patient's airway.
    - True o
    - False

11. In the total laryngectomy procedure, the surgeon creates a new airway.
    - True o
    - False

12. Each neoplasm of thelarynx creates a distinct sound, enabling accurate acoustic diagnosis.
    - True
    - False o

13.   The vocal fold produce a complex sound.
                  True ○
                  False
14.   Subglottic air pressure is related to vocal loudness.
                  True ○
                  False
15.   Giral are most prone to develop vocal nodules.
                  True
                  False ○
16.   A polyp is a benign neoplasm.
                  True ○
                  False
17.   Voice therapy may involve psychological counseling skills.
                  True ○
                  False
18.   Surgical treatment may completely eliminate a voice problem.
                  True ○
                  False
19.   A person with a voice disorder should be seen (or have been seen) by a physician.
                  True ○
                  False
20.   Voice therapy may involve increasing vocal loudness.
                  True ○
                  False
21.   Voice building is a simple short process.
                  True
                  False ○
22.   Neoplasms of the vocal folds may cause the voice to sound "breathy."
                  True ○
                  False
23.   Hypernasality may be a congenital problem.
                  True ○
                  False
24.   An artificial larynx may generate sound with pulmonary air pressure.
                  True ○
                  False
25.   Following trauma, a stent can support thelaryngeal cartilages while they heal.
                  True ○
                  False

Multiple Choice

1.   Poor or unplesant voice quality is called:
                  a.   dysphonia ○
                  b.   telephonia
                  c.   carcinoma
                  d.   aphonia
2.   A sliding change in pitch without audible break is called a:
                  a.   vibrato
                  b.   glissando
                  c.   glycerine
                  d.   tremolo

3.   Edema lowers vocal pitch by:
        a.   increasing tension
        b.   iicreasing mass o
        c.   increasing subglottic pressure
        d.   all of the above

4.   Aphonia may be caused by:
        a.   disease
        b.   psychological factors
        c.   paralysis
        d.   all of the above o

5.   What condition causes incomlete glottal closure through stiffening of te crocoarytenid joint?
        a.   anemia
        b.   paralysis
        c.   conversion reaction
        d.   anklyosis

6.   Mass lesions of the vocal folds produce which of the following changes?
        a.   alter their shape o
        b.   decrease their mass
        c.   increase their mobility
        d.   place them in the paramedian position

7.   Which of the following is a malignant neoplasm?
        a.   polyp
        b.   cyst
        c.   nodule
        d.   squamous cell carcinoma o

8.   Which condition can cause a voice disorder?
        a.   poor posture
        b.   lack of exercise
        c.   nasal twang
        d.   anemia o

9.   Isolation of a specific muscle group for relaxation is a technique of...
        a.   meditation
        b.   differential relaxation o
        c.   progressive relaxation
        d.   biofeedback

10. What term describes a surgically built tunnel connection the traches and the esophagus?
        a.   shunt (fistula) o
        b.   funnel (venturi)
        c.   chimney (tube)
        d.   window (fenestra)

11. At what point on the vocal fold margins do nodules usually form?
        a.   unilaterally at the cartilaginous portion of the folds
        b.   at the anterior juncture of the folds
        c.   bilaterally, in the midpoint of the membranous portion of the folds o
        d.   bilaterally, at the midpoint of the vocal folds

12. Which of the followong can create edema in the vocal folds?
        a.   pregnancy
        b.   allergic reactions
        c.   vocal abuse
        d.   all of the above o

13. What is the most common age for papillomata to form?
    a. six months to one year
    b. one ear to two years
    c. four years to six years o
    d. eight years to fifteen years
14. Which of the following may cause a laryngeal web?
    a. surgery
    b. injury
    c. congenital factors
    d. all of the above o
15. Most resonance disorders may be characterized by...
    a. breathiness
    b. nasal twang
    c. hyper- or hypo-nasality
    d. aphonia
16. What is the most ubiquitous electrical aid to voice diagnosis?
    a. a laryngeal mirror
    b. a sound recorder
    c. a sound spectrograph
    d. a boom box
17. Which childhood personality is associated with vocal abuse?
    a. shy, quiet, iterested in board games
    b. musically gifted, amiable, interested in pleasing the teacher
    c. dull, listless, interested in clothes
    d. competitive, aggressive, interested in sports o
18. Which of the following is part of madical intervention in voice therapy?
    a. hyperventilation
    b. relaxation
    c. finding optimum pitch
    d. Psychiatry o
19. Which of the folowing is part of direct intervention in voice therapy?
    a. Psychiatry
    b. avoiding polluting atmospheres
    c. regulation of breathing o
    d. creation of a P-E segment
20. Which of the following is part of an environmental approach to therapy
    a. reducing the amount of yelling and singing o
    b. excision of the nodules
    c. relaxation
    d. voice training
21. What is the physical relationship of the trachea to the esophagus?
    a. the trachea is posterior to the esophagus
    b. the trachea is anterior to the esophagus o
    c. the trachea is lateral to the esophagus
    d. the trachea is inferior to the esophagus

Answers to Self Test Chapter Nine

The Fluency Disorder of Stuttering

Peter R. Ramig and George H. Shames

True/False

1. Stuttering is simply a matter of repetitions of whole and part words.
        True
        False o
2. There appears to be no familial pattern in stuttering behavior
        True
        False o
3. The listener plays a role in the determination of whether or not dysfluency is a disorder.
        True o
        False
4. Most cases of stuttering start in the preschool years.
        True o
        False
5. The longer a stuttering problem exists, the more likely it is that associated emotional problems will develop.
        True o
        False
6. People who stutter may find that whispering reduces their symptoms.
        True o
        False
7. Monozygotic twins show a smaller percentage of stuttering in both children.
        True
        False o
8. Stuttering and cluttering are two names for the same disorder.
        True
        False o
9. Stutterers may experience greater difficulties when telling jokes.
        True o
        False
10. Recent evidence has largely refuted cerebral dominance theories of stuttering causation.
        True
        False o
11. There is little doubt that stuttering runs in families.
        True o
        False
12. At least some overt stuttering behavior as been controlled empirically by operant conditioning.
        True o
        False
13. Parents should view dysfluency in children between two and one half and three and one half years of age with great alarm.
        True
        False o

14. Stuttering intervention begun at an early age has a good success record.
    True ○
    False
15. Visible muscular tension while speaking is a normal sign.
    True
    False ○
16. The most valid and reliable assessment procedures are based on direct observation
    True ○
    False
17. Fluency shaping involves modification of stuttering moments.
    True
    False ○
18. Boys who stutter outnumber girls who stutter by a ratio of 4:1.
    True ○
    False
19. Stuttering therapy for preschool children may involve direct intervention.
    True ○
    False
20. Wingate defined stuttering to include the presence of emotional states.
    True
    False ○
21. Systematic desensitization teaches the stutterer to do something that competes with his anxiety about speaking.
    True ○
    False
22. Success in treatment means no relapses.
    True
    False ○
23. Counseling appears to be a necessary component of the total clinical management of stuttering.
    True ○
    False
24. Systematic desensitization is a technique based on the orientation that stuttering is conditioned.
    True ○
    False
25. Experimentation has revealed that stuttering can be prevented.
    True
    False ○

Multiple Choice

1. Which of the following is *NOT* one of Wingate's components of stuttering?
    a. presence of emotion
    b. disruptions of speech fluency
    c. accessory struggle and tension
    d. syntactic reversals ○
2. Which of the following characterize people who clutter?
    a. precocious language development
    b. incomplete utterances ○
    c. echolalia
    d. circumlocution

3. Which of the following did Goldman (1967) report regarding cultural differences in stuttering?
   a. More females stutter than males
   b. Japanese Americans have a low incidence of stuttering when they speak English.
   c. Twice as many African American males stutter as do African American Females. o
   d. British Americans place more speaking anxiety on their children.

4. Which of the following is an overt symptom of stuttering?
   a. repetitions
   b. absence of sound
   c. prolongations of sounds
   d. all of the above o

5. Which of the following conditions may reduce the severity of stuttering?
   a. singing o
   b. talking on the telephone
   c. telling a joke
   d. speaking to authority figures

6. According to surveys, which child is most likely to stutter?
   a. a monozygotic male twin who's twin brother stutters and who has a family history of stuttering. o
   b. a child with delayed language onset.
   c. a child with poor dentition who speaks two languages
   d. an African American male

7. Which cerebral hemisphere to proponents of the "Cerebral Dominance" theory of stuttering causation posit is dominant?
   a. left
   b. right
   c. both
   d. neither o

8. "Neurotic" theories suggest that...
   a. stuttering is a well-integrated, purposeful defense against some threatening idea. o
   b. whispering is a way to hide a stutterer's emotions.
   c. the telephone is protection from direct contact with others.
   d. most young children exhibit dysfluent speech.

9. The one true cause of stuttering is...
   a. lack of cerebral dominance
   b. conditioned behavior
   c. neurophysiologic breakdown
   d. unknown o

10. According to Sheehan's "approach-avoidance" construct, people who stutter have their anxieties reduced by..
    a. remaining silent
    b. speaking
    c. either speaking or remaining silent o
    d. stuttering

11. According to a survey by Bloodstein (1995) regarding incidence of stuttering in different countries, in which group did the United States fall?
    a. countries with substantially less stuttering o
    b. countries with an average amount of stuttering
    c. countries with substantially more stuttering
    d. countries with no stuttering

12. Which of the following statements best characterizes a child in Bloodstein's stuttering developmental "Phase 2"?
    a. occasional repetitions of initial words or syllables, little reaction
    b. chronic stutterer at times of excitement but doesn't care o
    c. occasionally reacts to stuttering with irritation
    d. stuttering regarded with fearful anticipation

13. According to Curlee and Van Riper how many dysfluencies constitute stuttering?
    a. repetitions in 1% of words uttered
    b. any prolongations and hesitations in 1% of words uttered
    c. prolongations longer than one second on 2% or more of words uttered o
    d. all of the above

14. According to Ramig (1990) which of the following is/are considered to be warning signals for a child exhibiting dysfluent speech?
    a. imprecise speech articulation
    b. avoidance of speech o
    c. self talk during play
    d. jargon early in speech development

15. Which is the goal of "Fluency-Shaping" therapy?
    a. inhibit anxiety with counter conditioned relaxation
    b. establish left cerebral hemisphere dominance
    c. teach acceptance of the problem
    d. demonstrate ways to increase fluency and replace stuttering

16. What kind of therapy model does "Reciprocal Inhibition" fit?
    a. fluency shaping
    b. modification therapy
    c. parental training
    d. delayed auditory feedback

17. Which of the following is a fluency-shaping treatment?
    a. changing parent-child interactions
    b. psychological therapy
    c. delayed auditory feedback o
    d. reciprocal inhibition

18. Researchers (Yaruss and Conture, 1995) have suggested that a parent may be speaking to fast if his/her rate of speech is...
    a. faster than that of the child
    b. two syllables per second faster than that of the child o.
    c. ten syllables per second faster than that of the child
    d. it depends on the language spoken by parent and child

19. Which of the following was a therapy approach of old?
    a. putting stones in the mouth
    b. oral surgery
    c. waving one hand in the air
    d. all of the above o

20. Which of the following do all therapy approaches for advanced stutterers have in common?
    a. self hypnosis
    b. focus on machinery
    c. imagery
    d. changing quality of interpersonal relationships o

21. Which of the following is maintenance activity?
    a. reinforcement by family and friends for fluency in non-clinical speech activities
    b. self-rating
    c. behavioral contracting
    d. all of the above o

22. Which is a necessary component of total clinical case management in stuttering?
     a. fluency-shaping
     b. metronome conditioned speech
     c. counseling
     d. delayed auditory feedback
23. Continued emission of target behaviors established during therapy is called...
     a. maintenance o
     b. counseling
     c. fluency-shaping
     d. reciprocal inhibition
24. What has research demonstrated about prevention of stuttering?
     a. Prevention depends on the severity of stuttering.
     b. Prevention of stuttering has not been demonstrated empirically. o
     c. Stuttering is the most preventable speech disorder
     d. One out of ten children who stutter could have been prevented from doing so.
25. Variations in treatment are partly functions of...
     a. a random choice
     b. the parents' ability to pay
     c. theoretical definition and perception of the problem o
     d. ASHA recommendations

True/False

1.   Sound waves travel in all directions from the source.
        True o
        False
2.   Amplitude is the number of compressions and rarefactions in a given time.
        True
        False o
3.   The amount of particle displacement is amplitude.
        True o
        False
4.   Frequency is measured in Hertz.
        True o
        False
5.   The decibel scale is named after Alexander Graham Bell.
        True o
        False
6.   Most natural sounds are pure tones.
        True
        False o
7.   The fundamental frequency of vowels in a speech wave is the frequency of the speaker's Glottic cycle (vocal fold vibration).
        True o
        False
8.   The first and second formants usually provide enough information to make vowels intelligible.
        True o
        False
9.   Impaired perception of prosodic spec elements may result in *deaf speech*.
        True o
        False
10. Most disorders of the outer ear cause significant hearing loss.
        True
        False o
11. Only the mother's ingestion of drugs can affect the unborn child.
        True
        False o

12. The middle ear plays a crucial role in sound localization.
   - True
   - False ○
13. The ossiclces are structures of the inner ear.
   - True
   - False ○
14. The inner ear serves two biological functions..
   - True ○
   - False
15. The *ear drum* is the entire middle ear.
   - True ○
   - False
16. Speech discrimination is measured with an SRT.
   - True
   - False ○
17. Some genetically based hearing disorders are not visible until later in life.
   - True ○
   - False
18. Hearing threshold refers to the softest sound which can be perceived 100% of the time.
   - True
   - False ○
19. ASL has the same syntax as General American English.
   - True
   - False ○
20. Pure tone audiometry results are always reliable.
   - True
   - False ○
21. An ABR is a form of hearing test.
   - True
   - False ○
22. The tympanogram measures thresholds for pure tones.
   - True
   - False ○
23. Implants may be placed directly into the brain stem.
   - True ○
   - False
24. For most people, a sound of about 85 dB SL l. will elicit a stapedial reflex.
   - True ○
   - False
25. Research suggested that deaf children who are fluent in ASL and English show superior achievement.
   - True ○
   - False

Multiple Choice

1. A crayon inserted in the external ear canal can result in what type of hearing loss?
   - a. conductive ○
   - b. sensorineural
   - c. mixed
   - d. central

2. ANSI established normal hearing level thresholds for pure tones at:
    a. 0 dB SL HL o
    b. 50 dB SL SPL
    c. variable, depending on the tone frequency.
    d. measured electronically

3. Audiologists refer to the area of an audiogram within which most speech frequencies and intensities are located as the...
    a. sensorineural zone
    b. talking area
    c. speech banana o
    d. speech fruit cocktail

4. Pure tone audiometry assesses...
    a. the type of hearing loss o
    b. stapedial reflex
    c. middle ear function
    d. speech discrimination

5. Normal pure tone hearing thresholds are in what range?
    a. 0-5 dB SL HL
    b. 10-15 dB SL HL o
    c. 0-10%
    d. IV-V dB SL re:.0002 dynes/cm³

6. What happens to middle ear impedance when there is fluid in the tympanum?
    a. It increases. o
    b. It decreases.
    c. It remains unchanged.
    d. It drains the fluid from the tympanic cavity.

7. Which type of tympanogram is normal in Jerger's (1970) nomenclature?
    a. Type A o
    b. Type B
    c. Type C
    d. Type D

8. Which of the following factors are chief determinants of hearing loss implications for an individual
    a. age of onset
    b. type of loss
    c. degree of loss
    d. all of the above o

9. What disease causes growth of bone in the oval window?
    a. measles
    b. endolymph
    c. cerebral palsy
    d. otosclerosis o

10. What causes atresia of the external ear canal?
    a. trauma
    b. otitis media
    c. gestation problems o
    d. ossicular discontinuity

11. A postnatal cause of hearing loss due to damage in the inner ear is:
    a. atresia
    b. otitis media
    c. rubeola
    d. all of the above o

431

12. Pure tone audiometry...
    a. uses involuntary responses
    b. uses voluntary responses ○
    c. is passive
    d. uses tuning forks
13. A person with a high frequency hearing loss would encounter the greatest difficulty perceiving:
    a. /a/
    b. /s/ ○
    c. /e/
    d. /m/
14. Zero decibels "Hearing Level" means...
    a. there is no sound.
    b. the intensity at which normal hearers can barely hear the sound. ○
    c. the listener has a hearing impairment.
    d. the frequency is neutral.
15. In sensorineural hearing loss, what is the usual comparison between air and bone conduction thresholds?
    a. Air conduction thresholds are lower than bone conduction thresholds.
    b. Air conduction thresholds are higher than bone conduction thresholds.
    c. Air conduction thresholds are within 10 dB SL of bone conduction thresholds. ○
    d. There are no bone conduction thresholds.
16. If a hearing loss occurs before the development of language it is said to be a:
    a. prelinguistic loss ○
    b. postlinguistic loss
    c. both of the above
    d. neither of the above
17. Which of the following is a *prosthesis?*
    a. hearing aid
    b. dental caps
    c. temporal bone stimulators
    d. all of the above ○
18. Which type of hearing loss is most readily curable?
    a. sensorineural
    b. cochlear
    c. conductive ○
    d. none of the above
19. A sound made up of multiple frequencies is said to be...
    a. complex ○
    b. pure
    c. complicated
    d. central
20. Infection of the middle ear is called...
    a. Meniere's disease
    b. Presbycusis
    c. Otitis externa
    d. Otitis media ○
21. How are neonates in medical distress identified?
    a. tattooing
    b. placement on the waiting list
    c. placement on the high-risk registry ○
    d. they are wrapped in purple p.j.'s

22. What is the most common complaint patients have about their hearing?
  a. They feel dizzy.
  b. They have difficulty hearing speech. ○
  c. They hear ringing in their ears.
  d. They have difficulty speaking.
23. What stimuli comprise most word recognition lists?
  a. sentences
  b. multisyllabic words
  c. bisyllabic words
  d. monosyllabic word ○
24. How long after stimulus presentation do auditory brainstem responses occur?
  a. within the first ten milliseconds ○
  b. after ten seconds
  c. not until one second has passed
  d. when the patient raises his/her hand
25. Which of the following is a type of hearing aid?
  a. AGC
  b. CIC ○
  c. ASL
  d. dB

Answers to Self Test Chapter Eleven

Cleft Palate

Betty Jane McWilliams and Mary Anne Witzel

True/False

1.   Structures of the face and palate fuse between the sixth and twelfth weeks of gestation.
         True o
         False
2.   A perceptive parent can encourage communication better than a certified speech-language pathologist.
         True o
         False
3.   All oral clefts are easily detected by visual inspection.
         True
         False o
4.   Several researchers have described a "Cleft Palate Personality."
         True
         False o
5.   Most infants with palatal clefts also have middle ear pathology..
         True o
         False
6.   Most children with complete clefts are also mentally retarded.
         True
         False o
7.   Males are more likely to have clefts than are females.
         True o
         False
8.   Orientals have a higher incidence of clefts than Blacks.
         True o
         False
9.   A cleft palate cannot occur without a cleft of the lip.
         True
         False o
10.   Syndromes of congenital malformations are phenotypic expressions of genotypic traits.
         True o
         False
11.   Articulation secondary to velopharyngeal incompetence are the ones we worry about most.
         True o
         False
12.   Negative intraoral air pressure is required for normal nursing.
         True o
         False
13.   The tensor veli palatini muscles play a partial role in eustachian tube function.
         True o
         False

14. Success of initial surgery is usually doubtful.
      True
      False o
15. Children with clefts talk more than other children.
      True
      False o
16. Language differences in children with clefts are less marked at later ages.
      True o
      False
17. Visible nasal air escape is observed with a mirror.
      True o
      False
18. When a speaker tries to valve with the nostrils, the result is a facial grimace
      True o
      False
19. Hypernasality is the likely result of enlarged adenoids.
      True
      False o
20. An opening from the palate into the nose is called an oral-nasal fistula
      True o
      False
21. The sibilants are most affected by velopharyngeal incompetence.
      True o
      False
22. A high narrow palate with excessive maxillary tissue is likely to be present in Apert's syndrome.
      True o
      False
23. Surgical correction of the velopharyngeal valve will eliminate articulation errors.
      True
      False o
24. Nasometry reveals nasal air flow problems.
      True
      False o
25. A prosthodontist specially designs speech aids for the individual patient.
      True o
      False

Multiple Choice

1. What kind of vocal tract resonance results when an anteriorly blocked nasal cavity is coupled with the rest of the vocal tract?
      a. hyponasal
      b. hypernasal
      c. hypo-hyper nasal
      d. cul de sac o
2. A submucous cleft is...
      a. easily observed with a mirror
      b. caused by trauma to the roof of the mouth
      c. a true muscular cleft o
      d. isolated in the upper lip

436

3.	Which of the following groups have the highest incidence of clefts?
	a.	females
	b.	Blacks
	c.	Caucasians
	d.	Orientals o

4.	What term describes defects of the head and face.
	a.	Teratology
	b.	Craniofacial abnormalities o
	d.	Syndactyly
	e.	Esophoria

5.	Which of the following techniques can help a baby with a cleft nurse successfully?
	a.	placing the baby in a supine position
	b.	early switching to a cup
	c.	holding the baby upright o
	d.	feeding with the baby in a prone position

6.	Which of the following may be the basis for speech articulation problems in children with clefts.
	a.	maturational lags
	b.	dental anomalies
	c.	hearing loss
	d.	all of the above o

7.	If the dental arch is involved in a cleft, how is the cleft classified?
	a.	isolated
	b.	complete o
	c.	submucous
	d.	lip

8.	Which phonemes are most likely to be produced with some nasal air escape?
	a.	vowels
	b.	glides
	c.	fricatives o
	d.	plosives

9.	What speech characteristic is most commonly associated with velopharyngeal incompetence?:
	a.	cul de sac resonance
	b.	hypernasality o
	c.	hyponasality
	d.	denasality

10.	Which articulatory compensatory posture is common among speakers with clefts?
	a.	lisping
	b.	labialization
	c.	tongue backing o
	d.	tongue fronting

11.	What phonatory behavior is thought to cause vocal problems among people with clefts?
	a.	retention of subglottic air o
	b.	using too high a vocal pitch
	c.	loud speech
	d.	speaking on supplemental air

12.	What are the medical therapies for middle-ear disease?
	a.	aeration tubes
	b.	myringotomy
	c.	antibiotics
	d.	all of the above o

13. Which visualization technique is the most inclusive?
    a. cephalometry
    b. cinefluoroscopy
    c. multiview videofluoroscopy ○
    d. nasendoscopy
14. One estimate of the prevalence of cleft disorders in the black population ranges from:
    a. 1 in 3000 births ○
    b. 1 in 500 births
    c. 1 in 750 births
    d. 1 in 1200 births
15. Which surgical procedure is used to improve velopharyngeal valving?
    a. tracheostomy
    b. myringotomy
    c. tonsillectomy/adenoidectomy
    d. pharyngeal flap ○
16. Which professional creates dental appliances?
    a. Orthodontist
    b. Prosthodontist ○
    c. Dentist
    d. Velodontist
17. The least invasive articulation disorder attributable to velopharyngeal incompetence is:
    a. reduced intraoral pressure on sibilants ○
    b. reduced intraoral pressure on plosives
    c. glottal stops
    d. pharyngeal fricatives
18. An opening from the palate into the nasal cavity is called a...
    a. cranial fossa
    b. pharyngotympanic tube
    c. oral-nasal fistula ○
    d. bifid uvula
19. Nasal semivowel production is likely to be distorted when the speaker is...
    a. hyponasal ○
    b. hypernasal
    c. aphasic
    d. dysphagic
20. The nasometer measures
    a. turbulence
    b. nasal air emission
    c. velopharyngeal insufficiency
    d. nasal resonance ○
21. What can multiview videofluoroscopy show?
    a. presence or absence of an opening between the oral and nasal cavities during speech
    b. an estimate about the size of the opening
    c. the shape of the orifice
    d. all of the above ○
22. Which is a disadvantage of nasendoscopy?
    a. it is expensive
    b. it is invasive ○
    c. it does not involve radiation
    d. it can be used by a speech pathology aide

23. What is an alternative surgical treatment to pharyngeal flap?
    a. implant o
    b. laryngeal flap
    c. lingual frenum section
    d. prosthesis
24. After surgical treatment, gross articulatory errors are treated with...
    a. prosthesis
    b. speech therapy o
    c. orthodontia
    d. no treatment is required
25. When should correction of major dental anomalies should take place?
    a. before speech therapy o
    b. during speech therapy
    c. after speech therapy
    d. the timing is not crucial

True/False

1. More brain area is devoted to control of the speech musculature than for the lower extremities.
    > True o
    > False

2. Dysarthria of speech refers to difficulty to formulate spoken language units.
    > True
    > False o

3. Neurogenic speech disorders can be caused by neoplasms.
    > True o
    > False

4. Race or ethnic factors play no role in nervous system damage.
    > True
    > False o

5. A good short term goal for modification of respiration is producing a pressure of 5mm of water for five sec.
    > True o
    > False

6. Sometimes braces of slings can increase the firmness of the speech production system's foundation.
    > True o
    > False

7. Neurogenic communication disorders may affect the spinal or cranial nerves of the peripheral nervous system.
    > True o
    > False

8. Speech movement depends solely on muscular strength.
    > True
    > False o

9. Articulatory accuracy in volitional speech is more difficult for the patient with apraxia.
    > True o
    > False

10. Firearms-related injury is the leading cause of head trauma.
    > True
    > False o

11. Dysphagia is always accompanied by dysarthria of speech.
    > True
    > False o

12. The first thing a clinician must decide is what type of dysarthria is present.
    > True
    > False o

13. The patient with dysarthria frequently gropes for an articulatory target.
   - True
   - False ○
14. Patients with dysarthria usually have no difficulty initiating speech.
   - True ○
   - False
15. Approximately one in five Americans has some kind of neurological or communication disorder
   - True ○
   - False
16. The most prevalent cause of neurotoxicity is alcohol and drug abuse.
   - True ○
   - False
17. Lesions located in small critical brain areas can produce severe impairment.
   - True ○
   - False
18. Apraxia can affect the execution of non-speech movements.
   - True ○
   - False
19. Therapeutic goals for modifying prosody are only appropriate for patients with apraxia.
   - True
   - False ○
20. Hypokinetic dysarthria is a result of Parkinson's disease
   - True ○
   - False
21. Traumatic brain injuries affect more people over forty years of age than it does any other age group.
   - True
   - False ○
22. Speech-language pathologists are concerned only with speech intelligibility.
   - True
   - False ○
23. Spastic dysarthria is associated with brainstem disorders.
   - True
   - False ○
24. Disorders of multiple motor systems can result in mixtures of several dysarthria types.
   - True ○
   - False
25. Experience will enable the clinician to classify dysarthria type in any case.
   - True
   - False ○

Multiple Choice

1. Which of the following is a neurogenic communication disorder?
   a. oral apraxia
   b. literal paraphasia
   c. dysarthria
   d. all of the above ○

2.   Speech intelligibility is negatively influenced by...
       a.   involuntary movements
       b.   inadequate range of movement o
       c.   excessive rate
       d.   uninhibited activity of intact nervous system parts
3.   Which of the following is a characteristic of apraxia?
       a.   frequent substitution errors o
       b.   simplification of consonant clusters
       c.   consistent quality of production
       d.   no difficulty in speech initiation
4.   What term describes the relatively constant state of muscular contraction?
       a.   strength
       b.   timing
       c.   organization
       d.   tone o
5.   Which of the seven point-places affects prosody?
       a.   1
       b.   2
       c.   4 -7
       d.   all o
6.   What is the principle feature of resonance that a clinician assesses?
       a.   harshness
       b.   pharyngeal tension
       c.   oral-nasal resonance balance o
       d.   oral-buccal resonance
7.   Motor impairment of which speech system components most affects intelligibility?
       a.   articulatory o
       b.   respiratory
       c.   resonance
       d.   phonatory
8.   Which dimensions of speech are affected by dysarthria?
       a.   content and relevance
       b.   intelligibility and bizarreness o
       c   syntax and phonology
       d.   pragmatics and initiation
9.   Which of the following may be a cause of neurogenic speech disorders?
       a.   trauma
       b.   cerebral palsy
       c.   snake bites
       d.   all of the above o
10.   The term *flaccid dysarthria* is associated with:
       a.   marked hypotonicity o
       b.   marked hypertonicity
       c.   marked tremor
       d.   none of the above
11.   Ataxia is a disorder of:
       a.   the cerebral cortex
       b.   the brainstem
       c.   the peripheral nervous system
       d.   the cerebellum o

443

12. Variability of production patterns is a characteristic of ...
    a. apraxia ○
    b. ataxia
    c. hypokinetic dysarthria
    d. spastic dysarthria
13. The Point-Place System assesses valves in which direction?
    a. superior to inferior
    b. lateral to medial
    c. central to peripheral
    d. inferior to superior ○
14. If a native language speaking patient has a foreign accent, it may be a sign of...
    a. pseudoforeign accent ○
    b. pseudobulbar palsy
    c. pseudomonas bacillus
    d. pseudolinguistic prosodius
15. A child who demonstrates increased errors as utterance length increases may have what disorder?
    a. dysarthria
    b. aphasia
    c. developmental apraxia ○
    d. phonological disorder
16. What is the first question the assessing clinician must answer?
    a. does a significant problem exist? ○
    b. what is the nature of the impairment?
    c. how handicapping is the condition?
    d. are some language functions intact?
17. What activity does integral stimulation treatment involve?
    a. modification of sitting posture
    b. deriving one phonetic posture from another, similar one
    c. modeling of speech postures ○
    d. application of surface electrodes to the fixed articulator
18. Which of the following long-term objectives applies when return to minimal speech function is not possible?
    a. train in use of artificial larynx
    b. return to normal speech function
    c. train in resonance modification
    d. train in use of alternative communicative device ○
19. "Tapping" might be an activity in what kind treatment?
    a. modification of phonation
    b. modification of resonance
    c. modification of articulation
    d. modification of prosody ○
20. The purpose of counseling with patients who have neurogenic communicative disorders in includes...
    a. conveyance of information
    b. provision of emotional support
    c. improve environmental communication variables
    d. all of the above ○
21. The development of progressively more difficult speech tasks involves what strategy?
    a. developing task continua ○
    b. drill
    c. the points along the Nile
    d. Ethel Merman therapy

22. Which type of therapy requires the consultation of other professionals?
    a. modification of respiration for speech
    b. modification of posture ○
    c. modification of articulation
    d. modification of prosody

Answers to Self Test Chapter Thirteen

Aphasia and Related Disorders

Carol S. Swindell, Audrey L. Holland and O.M. Reinmuth

True/False

1. The most common cause of aphasia is "stroke."
    True o
    False

2. Right hemispheres lesions can affect the way a patient uses speech prosody.
    True o
    False

3. Self-concept may be jeopardized as a result of aphasia.
    True o
    False

4. The right hemisphere contains the centers for language function in most individuals.
    True
    False o

5. Wernicke's aphasia is on of the *nonfluent* aphasias.
    True
    False o

6. Aphasia has been caused by damage to subcortical structures.
    True o
    False

7. Aphasia in children is treated the same as aphasia in adults.
    True
    False o

8. Visual impulses generated n the right eye are processed only by the left cerebral hemisphere.
    True
    False o

9. Loss of vision in half of the visual field is called quadrantal anopsia.
    True
    False o

10. Lesions of the right hemisphere sometimes produce unilateral *neglect*.
    True o
    False

11. The inability to recall the names of objects is *agrammatism*.
    True
    False o

12. Initiation of speech is generally left unimpaired in nonfluent aphasias.
    True
    False o

13. Damage to Wernicke's area produces difficulties on comprehending speech.
    True o
    False

14. Substitution of in-semantic-class words, such as "knife" for "fork" are called phonemic or literal paraphasias.
    True
    False o

15. *Broca's aphasia* is characterized by sparse, slow, labored speech.
    True o
    False

16. Some recovery from aphasia is likely to occur after a few months, with or without therapy.
    True o
    False

17. The majority of studies are equivocal regarding the effectiveness of speech therapy for aphasia.
    True
    False o

18. Fluent aphasias are most commonly the result of lesions in the posterior part of the dominant cerebral hemisphere.
    True o
    False

19. Children with acquired aphasia rarely demonstrate any significant degree of recovery.
    True
    False o

20. Formal evaluation is most useful immediately following a cerebral injury or as soon as possible.
    True
    False o

21. Destruction of the visual cortex of one hemisphere would result in hemianopsia.
    True o
    False

22. *Reauditorizaton* is a term that describes the reorganization of auditory processes during recovery from aphasia.
    True o
    False

23. The *Porch Index of Communicative Abilities* is the only aphasia instrument that seeks to predict recovery potential.
    True o
    False

24. Melodic intonation therapy is a carefully sequenced series of activities that helps the patient reestablish representational behavior through gestures.
    True
    False o

25. We do not know how the brain capitalizes on therapy activities.
    True o
    False

Multiple Choice

1. Most children acquire aphasia as a result of...
    a. developmental delays
    b. neonatal hypoxia
    c. head injury or diseases o
    d. lack of stimulation

2. Which of the following language disturbances most often results from brain damage in the posterior speech areas?
    a. fluent speech
    b. auditory comprehension difficulties o
    c. slow, labored speech
    d. motor programming deficits
3. In which aphasia pattern is almost normal language marred by word retrieval difficulties?
    a. Conduction aphasia
    b. Broca's aphasia
    c. Wernicke's aphasia
    d. Anomic aphasia o
4. What type of paralysis results from damage to the motor cortex of one cerebral hemisphere?
    a. hemiplegia o
    b. diplegia
    c. athetosis
    d. quadriplegia
5. Which of the following is a type of "stroke?"
    a. embolism
    b. hemorrhage
    c. thrombosis
    d. all of the above o
6. If a patient presents with unilateral right hemiplegia, to which cerebral hemisphere might we infer damage?
    a. right hemisphere
    b. left hemisphere o
    c. both hemispheres
    d. neither hemisphere
7. Why is any paralysis combined with aphasia most often a right hemiplegia?
    a. Aphasia most often results from damage to the left cerebral hemisphere. o
    b. Hemiplegia is a language disturbance following a stroke.
    c. Hemiplegia most often involves the ipsilateral hemisphere.
    d. Strokes are the most common cause of aphasia.
8. Which of the following is not an aphasia treatment approach?
    a. Melodic Intonation Therapy
    b. Reauditorization
    c. Visual Action Therapy
    d. Neurodevelopmental Treatment o
9. Which of the following is most true about aphasia?
    a. It is a speech disorder.
    b. It is a breakdown in the ability to process the symbols of language o
    c. It has gradual onset.
    d. It is a learned condition
10. The use of *Stereotypes* is most associated with:
    a. Broca's aphasia
    b. Wernicke's aphasia
    c. Global aphasia o
    d. Mixed aphasia
11. Interruption of blood flow through the left cerebral artery in adulthood is most likely to produce which disorder?
    a. left unilateral neglect
    b. aphasia o
    c. flaccid dysarthria
    d. left hemiplegia

12. Which area of the brain is of most interest to aphasiologists?
   a. pons
   b. cortex o
   c. basal ganglia
   d. corpus callosum

13. Which of the following is a *nonfluent* aphasic syndrome?
   a. Wernicke's
   b. Conduction
   c. Transcortical Sensory
   d. Global o

14. One commonly-held theory about the jargon of Wernicke's aphasia supposes that...
   a. The patient has paralysis of the muscles of speech articulation.
   b. The patient has difficulty comprehending her own speech. o
   c. The patent has difficulty with word retrieval.
   d. The patient has difficulty programming the muscles of speech.

15. Which of the following mechanisms is most likely to produce focal cerebral deficits?
   a. stroke o
   b. closed head trauma
   c. diabetic coma
   d. anoxia

16. Which of the following is generally thought to be a *right* hemisphere function?
   a. word retrieval
   b. speech programing
   c. short term memory
   d. music appreciation o

17. The chronically aphasic patient is one...
   a. who continues to improve two months post onset.
   b. spontaneous recovery has reached a plateau . o
   c. has had a recent exacerbation .
   d. receives no further benefit from therapy.

18. Of the following tests of aphasia, which attempts to profile aphasic syndromes?
   a. Boston Diagnostic Aphasia Evaluation o
   b. Western Aphasia Battery
   c. Communicative Ability of Daily Living
   d. Porch Index of Communicative Abilities

19. Language behaviors that result from closed head trauma are:
   a. motor
   b. among generalized deficits o
   c. focused on a certain language modality
   d. focal language deficits

20. On the *Rancho Los Amigos Hospital's Levels of Cognitive Recovery Scale*, which level is the closest to independence?
   a. RLA 2
   b. RLA 5
   c. RLA 6
   d. RLA8 o

21. How have we inferred localization of cerebral cortical functions?
   a. experimental lesions in animals
   b. direct stimulation of human subjects' brains
   c. relating post mortem findings with case history data
   d. all of the above o

22. Damage to which of the following areas has the highest likelihood of producing nonfluent aphasia?
    a. Broca's area o
    b. the left occipital lobe
    c. Wernicke's area
    d. the right temporal-parietal juncture
23. How long post onset in the period during which most spontaneous changes in language deficits have occurred?
    a. 24 hours
    b. one week
    c. 30 days
    d. 60 days o
24. Which of the following is one purpose of all formal tests of language ability?
    a. measurement of patient's intelligence quotient
    b. disentangle the source of a patient's difficulty on a language task o
    c. profile the patient's aphasic syndrome
    d. predict recovery potential
25. In Wertz', *et al.* (1984a) study of aphasia treatment effectiveness how did the group that did not receive therapy for twelve weeks perform after twelve subsequent weeks of therapy?
    a. poorer than the groups that received therapy for the whole time
    b. better than the groups that received therapy for the whole time
    c. the same as the groups that received therapy the whole time o
    d. like they had never had aphasia

True/False

1. AAC intervention is only suitable for those who have acquired communication disorders.
   True
   False o

2. AAC use might replace a reason for challenging behavior in children.
   True o
   False

3. Augmentative devices are designed to communicate an entire message.
   True
   False o

4. Operational competence is not important in AAC intervention.
   True
   False o

5. American Indian hand talk uses a symbol system.
   True
   False o

6. Iconicity has been associated with learning success in mentally retarded individuals.
   True o
   False

7. Direct selection methods are those in which the possible choices are offered in sequence.
   True
   False o

8. One possible aided selection technique uses eye gaze to indicate a symbol on a clear acrylic board.
   True
   False o

9. In partner-assisted auditory scanning, the speakers partner speaks out the options on the array.
   True o
   False

10. Infants and toddlers are too young to derive benefit from AAC.
    True
    False o

11. Bliss symbols have a high degree of iconicity.
    True
    False o

12. Synthesized speech systems can produce virtually any message.
    True o
    False

13. Dedicated AAC devices are designed to perform functions beyond communication.
    True
    False o

453

14. Multimodal communication includes facial posture, facial expression and gestures in addition to the spoken signal.
    - True ○
    - False
15. A weakness of AAC devices is that they have poor figure-ground differential.
    - True
    - False ○
16. Learning that a symbol represents a referent is easier when they both exist in the same stimulus mode.
    - True ○
    - False
17. Graphic symbols have the advantage of permanency
    - True ○
    - False
18. The user's sensory capabilities are important in planning AAC strategy.
    - True ○
    - False
19. Social competence varies between cultural contexts.
    - True ○
    - False
20. The clinician is well-advised to obtain funding for a dedicated electronic alternative communication device for a patient with a temporary communicative disability.
    - True
    - False ○
21. The patent who cannot move his upper extremities is not a candidate for a dedicated AAC device.
    - True
    - False ○
22. Standardized assessments are perfectly suitable for rating cognitive functions in potential AAC users.
    - True
    - False ○
23. Some AAC users may attend college classes.
    - True ○
    - False
24. Digitized speech sounds more natural that synthesized speech.
    - True ○
    - False
25. Criteria-based assessments reduce the extent of information gathered to begin a particular intervention.
    - True ○
    - False
26. The potential AAC user's family may provide important information for planning intervention.
    - True ○
    - False
27. AAC devices can be programmed applications of the user's personal computer..
    - True ○
    - False

Multiple Choice

1. Aided AAC techniques require:
    - a. external equipment ○
    - b. picture boards
    - c. switching devices
    - d. no external equipment

2. Which of the following is an aspect of the AAC process?
    a. means to remember
    b. means to reproduce
    c. means to represent o
    d. means to relate
3. Which of the following is symbol system?
    a. American Indian Hand Talk
    b. Picsyms
    c. Lexigrams
    d. American Sign Language o
4. Unaided symbol systems...
    a. require an external device.
    b. attach one meaning to one symbol.
    c. are collections of ideograms.
    d. are rule-based and expressed with the speakers body. o
5. Communication devices that require external equipment are referred to as:
    a. aided devices o
    b. dedicated devices
    c. unaided devices
    d. none of the above
6. Which of the following symbols has the greatest amount of *iconicity?*
    a. a printed word
    b. a line drawing of the object o
    c. a spoken word
    d. a gesture
7. Which of the following statements is true regarding symbol systems?
    a. They have a greater representational range than symbol sets.
    b. They can represent abstract and concrete concepts equally well.
    c. They have their own linguistic rules.
    d. all of the above o
8. Symbol complexity (in Blissymbols) is...
    a. the number of lines used to make up the symbol o
    b. the number of meanings the symbol can have
    c. the degree of abstractness of the symbol
    d. the material of which the symbol is composed
9. Which of the following is a consideration for symbol selection?
    a. the cost
    b. culture of the potential speaker
    c. sensory demands
    d. all of the above o
10. The degree to which symbols seem different is called:
    a. complexity
    b. iconicity
    c. perceptual distinctness o
    d. all of the above
11. Which of the following concepts is concrete?
    a. love o
    b. dog
    c. man
    d. hat

12. Which of the following is a characteristic thought to affect symbol learning?
    a. iconicity
    b. complexity
    c. perceptual distinctness
    d. all of the above ○

13. Using a head stick to point to a symbol is an example of...
    a. unaided scanning
    b. aided direct selection ○
    c. unaided direct selection
    d. directed selection

14. Which type of scanning is the slowest and most cumbersome?
    a. linear scanning ○
    b. row-column scanning
    c. block scanning
    d. directed scanning

15. The user must stop the scanning with a switch in which type of scanning?
    a. linear scanning
    b. row-column scanning
    c. block scanning
    d. automatic scanning ○

16. Means to transmit refers to...
    a. the manner in which the communication partner receives the message ○
    b. the array of possible symbols used for communication.
    c. the type of scanning employed by the sender.
    d. how the individual chooses the symbols.

17. Which type of speech is a computer encoding phonemes through acoustic algorithms?
    a. synthesized speech ○
    b. digitized speech
    c. both of the above
    d. neither of the above

18. An advantage of synthesized speech is...
    a. high intelligibility
    b. low memory requirement ○
    c. high degree of naturalness
    d. ease in programming

19. An advantage of digitized speech is:
    a. low memory requirements
    b. great flexibility
    c. good quality signal ○
    d. unlimited number of possible messages

20. Adapted strategies that are called into play in the event of a communication breakdown are components of...
    a. linguistic competence.
    b. operational competence.
    c. social competence.
    d. strategic competence. ○

21. Social competence includes the communication skills of...:
    a. phonology
    b. sociolinguistics ○
    c. semantics
    d. tactical linguistics

22. A *feature matching* approach consists of...
    a. ensuring the patient will use the AAC device.
    b. matching users who have the same devices.
    c. matching therapists who share the same theoretical backgrounds.
    d. matching features of the AAC strategy or device with the needs of the client. ○

23. The ability of the client to comprehend the symbol system depends on which skills?
    a. cognitive and sensory ○
    b. dexterity and coordination
    c. social and pragmatic
    d. none of the above

24. Early use of AAC might be directed in which direction?
    a. increasing the child's self-talk
    b. increasing the child's participation in daily routines ○
    c. increasing the child's appreciation for electronic technology
    d. increasing the manual dexterity of the child

25. Which of the following disabilities may call for temporary use of AAC?
    a. dysarthria
    b. ALS
    c. cerebral palsy
    d. tracheostomy ○

26. In which assessment format is the client able to try several different AAC devices?
    a. center-based assessment ○
    b. maximum assessment
    c. naturalistic assessment
    d. standardized assessment

27. Examiners using commercial standardized tests in AAC assessment must remember what when interpreting results?
    a. Children become fatigued easily.
    b. The norm-references are no longer valid. ○
    c. Norm tables are grouped by age.
    d. Scores should be reported by using an AAC device.

28. Public law 101-336 protects...
    a. the civil rights of disabled individuals. ○
    b. racial hiring preferences.
    c. equal educational opportunity.
    d. the rights of clinicians in all disciplines.

Answers to Self Test Chapter Fifteen

Cerebral Palsy

James C. Hardy

True/False

1. The incidence of cerebral palsy is so low that special programs are not required.
    - True
    - False o

2. Cerebral palsy is caused only by hemorrhage in the brain
    - True
    - False o

3. Low birth weight is a common cause of cerebral palsy.
    - True
    - False o

4. Mental retardation rarely accompanies cerebral palsy.
    - True
    - False o

5. A distinguishing characteristic of cerebral palsy is that it is progressive.
    - True
    - False o

6. An estimate of the incidence of occurrence of cerebral palsy is 1.5-2 children per 1000 births.
    - True o
    - False

7. Spasticity is the most prevalent form of neuromotor dysfunction in cerebral palsy.
    - True o
    - False

8. Hypokinesia is not seen in cerebral palsy.
    - True o
    - False

9. Ataxia is a neuromotor dysfunction characterized by uninhibited stretch reflex.
    - True
    - False o

10. The term *athetosis* is being supplanted by the term *dyskinesia*.
    - True o
    - False

11. Dyskinesia is the most prevalent neuromotor dysfunction observed in cerebral palsy.
    - True
    - False o

12. Infants exhibit reflexive patterns similar to the movements of reptiles
    - True o
    - False

13.   Reflexes that hold our bodies upright depend, in part, upon the positions of our heads.
                    True o
                    False
14.   Spasticity is a mental condition associated with cerebral palsy.
                    True
                    False o
15.   A person with hemiplegia has paralysis of both lower extremities.
                    True
                    False o
16.   Developmental apraxia has been determined to be a frequent characteristic of cerebral palsy.
                    True
                    False o
17.   Sensations originate through activation of the central nervous system.
                    True
                    False o
18.   Dysprosody has no effect on communication efficiency.
                    True
                    False o
19.   The unique and distinguishing communication disorder of persons with cerebral palsy is dysarthria.
                    True o
                    False
20.   High frequency hearing loss is associated with damage to the developing brain.
                    True o
                    False
21.   Trauma is an infrequent cause of cerebral palsy.
                    True o
                    False
22.   For children with no potential of improving speech, dismissal from therapy is probably best for all involved.
                    True o
                    False
23.   With modern electronics, there is no longer any use for "low-tech" augmentative/alternative communication devices.
                    True
                    False o
24.   The motor disorders that accompany cerebral palsy are quite similar to those acquired by some people as adults.
                    True
                    False o
25.   Postural support systems are of little use in cases of cerebral palsy.
                    True
                    False o

Multiple Choice

1.   Cerebral palsy is essentially:
                    a.   a progressive neuromotor disorder.
                    b.   a progressive perceptual disorder
                    c.   a nonprogressive intellectual dysfunction
                    d.   a nonprogressive neuromotor disorder o

2. Which of the following may cause cerebral palsy?
   a. hemorrhage
   b. anoxia
   c. trauma
   d. all of the above o

3. The incidence of cerebral palsy is
   a. 1.5 children per 2,000 births
   b. 2 children per 1,500 births
   c. 1.5 to 2 children per 1000 births o
   d. 1.5 children per 1,500 births

4. The premature liver secretes a substance called
   a. jaundice
   b. bilirubin o
   c. hemoglobin
   d. substantia nigra

5. Which of the following neuromotor disorders is not sen in cerebral palsy?
   a. hypotonia o
   b. spasticity
   c. dyskinesia
   d. ataxia

6. Which of the following muscular conditions is related to the individual's emotional state?
   a. spasticity
   b. tension o
   c. hypotonicity
   d. athetosis

7. A generalized increase in muscle tone when considerable physical effort is exerted is called...
   a. athetosis
   b. chorea
   c. ataxia
   d. overflow o

8. The cerebellum is the part of the brain considered essential to...
   a. control of stretch reflex
   b. initiation of movement
   c. coordination of synergistic muscles o
   d. inhibition of movement

9. Hyperactivity of reflexes is characteristic of which form of neuromotor dysfunction?
   a. spasticity o
   b. dyskinesia
   c. ataxia
   d. hypokinesia

10. What term describes spastic involvement of the legs with little or no involvement of oral or upper extremity musculature?
    a. diplegia
    b. quadriplegia
    c. paraplegia o
    d. hemiplegia

11. What is the typical respiratory dysfunction in cerebra palsy?
    a. to much force in exhalation
    b. inhalatory stridor
    c. reduction in the amount of air inhalation and exhalation o
    d. low respiratory rate

461

12. What is the physician's role in management of cerebral palsy?
   a. establishment of initial diagnosis and monitoring health o
   b. evaluation of learning potential and adjustment patterns
   c. longitudinal observation of the child's communication behavior
   d. assist with the problems of upper extremity involvement and daily living

13. Which pioneering neurologist recognized subgroups within the diagnosis of cerebral palsy?
   a. Sigmund Freud o
   b. W.J. Little
   c. A. Gesell
   d.. K.L. Blackman

14. Which of the following occurs most infrequently in cerebral palsy?
   a. hypertonia
   b. flaccidity
   c. hypotonia
   d. ataxia o

15. As many as one third of patients who have spasticity or dyskinesia show signs of ...
   a. mixed type o
   b. chorea
   c. tremor
   d. ataxia

16. What is a likely developmental course for infantile reflexes in children with cerebral palsy?
   a. They disappear too early.
   b. They are retained and exaggerated. o
   c. They move to the lower extremity only
   d. They become more primitive.

17. What type of paralysis involves the upper and lower extremities of only one side of the body
   a. diplegia
   b. hemiplegia o
   c. quadriplegia
   d. paraplegia

18. Monotony of speech is a sign of...
   a. dysprosody. o
   b. respiratory dysfunction.
   c. hemiplegia
   d. imprecise consonant articulation.

19. Which Public Law prohibits discrimination against persons with disabilities?
   a. IDEA
   b. EEOC
   c. Affirmative Action
   d. ADA o

20. Which type of AAC device is probably best for individuals with limited intellectual abilities?
   a. digitized speech
   b. low-tech system o
   c. synthesized speech
   d. row-column scanning